A True St...
Stage IV P...

THE DAY
—— *the* ——
CANCER
QUIT

KRISTIE ANNE MAH

The Day The Cancer Quit
Published by Kristie Anne Mah
kristieannemah.com

For permissions contact **kam@kristieannemah.com**

Copyright© 2020 Kristie Anne Mah
All rights reserved. This book or any portion thereof may not be reproduced or used in any manner whatsoever without the express written permission of the publisher except for the use of brief quotations in a book review.

Cover & Interior Layout by: Serhat Özalp

Paperback ISBN: 9781777152727
Ebook ISBN: 9781777152710

*

Dedicated to God/the Universe- the source of infinite possibilities and healing, my parents for instilling in me the love to read and write, my true friends for their endless support, my husband for being my inspiration, and my children for teaching me to find the beauty in each and every day.

Contents

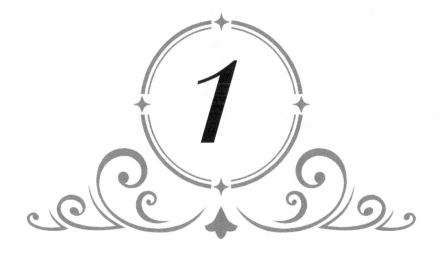

Chapter

HOW A NAME CAN MEAN SO MUCH

It was early spring, 2009, and while it was still chilly outside with frost settled in the corner of the windowpane, Terri and I were enjoying the warm sunlight streaming through our front window. It was just warm enough for me to take off my socks and ask for a much-needed footrest. I was, after all, 6 months pregnant with our first child, and was experiencing the typical restless legs and swollen feet.

"We really should discuss names," I said as I took a deep breath. "Baby will be here before we know it." Just at that moment, I felt a flutter and grabbed Terri's hands to feel the kick in my belly. "See—baby even wants us to decide a name right now," I teased.

After much conversation and tossing around of many ideas, Terri said he needed some inspiration. I wasn't sure exactly what that meant—a run, a green tea, a nap or some loud music. Moments later he returned with some magazines and started flipping through pages.

"Well," he said, "what about the name Maddox for a boy?"

"Yes, I like that one," I smiled. "Let's keep that on the maybe list."

"I have another one—I like the ring of Nixon for a boy as well."

"Agreed!" I smiled even bigger and sat up to rest my head on his shoulder. "Neither of those names resonate too much if this sweet baby is a girl though," I giggled.

We tossed around a few more names... Lucy, Samantha, Ariahna. I was starting to get tired and feeling like I needed a nap. Then just like that, it happened, with the flip of a page.

"What about Vienna?" he asked. "Vienna Ariahna?"

I didn't just like that name.

I didn't just love that name.

It was the name.

I cannot put into words the emotion I felt at that moment. Hearing those words took my breath away. I felt a little bit lightheaded and the hair on the back of my neck stood straight up. It was so intense I almost lost my balance as I flew off the couch.

I shouted, "Yes! Yes—that is the name. If baby is a girl, that is her name."

Looking back now, I know it was a message from God, the Universe giving me a sign... the epic truth of no coincidences. All of it aligning.

Other than marrying Terri, I had never felt so sure of anything in my entire life.

Our wonderful, beautiful baby boy was born in July 2009. We welcomed Nixon into our lives as a perfect bundle of joy. He was the happiest baby you could ever imagine; even if he woke at 3am he was grinning ear to ear. Full of life and love, to this day. He is still the most impeccable and amazing young man we could ever dream of having for a son.

Almost 2 years later to the day, we were blessed to welcome our second child into our family. The *million-dollar family,* we felt so fortunate to embrace a beautiful baby girl into our arms. So genuine and kind, her heart and passion for life were there from day one. She radiated warmth then and now, and her personality is contagious.

Without hesitation, we named her Vienna Ariahna. The name held power from the moment Terri spoke it that day we were sitting on the couch.

Little did I know then that Vienna's name had so much power for the story of our family. Not only is she our beautiful baby girl, but that Vienna would also be where we went to save Terri's life.

Vienna Ariahna—our daughter. Vienna, Austria—the city. No coincidences.

Even as I write this, I wonder how much more all of our lives would change and improve if we trusted God, the Universe and our intuition?

Mild Indigestion

Have you ever had those moments when you feel like you have been slapped so hard energetically that your insides are burning, your breath quickens, your head starts spinning and you feel like you are going to faint?

May 12th, 2017.

Terri came through the door from his checkup with the doctor explaining that his mild indigestion that used to come and go, was no longer leaving. They had done an ultrasound earlier in the week and noticed some hemangiomas on his liver but did not seem too worried. They sent him for a CT scan just to be sure. Our doctor, Dr. Manoji Wirasinghe, was incredible and absolutely on the ball. From the time of the checkup to the results of the CT was 5 days total. We will always have great appreciation for that expediency.

Since no one seemed concerned, I was not planning to attend his GP follow up appointment with him, instead spending the morning with Vienna before she went to kindergarten. Such precious moments with her were passing quickly.

That morning, long before he was supposed to attend the clinic, Terri received a phone call from the Endoscopy department. "We are so sorry to hear this news, and we would like to book you in right away for a scope and biopsy."

"What news?" Terri asked, shocked and bewildered.

Stumbling with her words, the nurse on the other end of the phone, apologetically and embarrassingly, asked Terri to call back once he had spoken to Dr. Wirasinghe.

In a daze, he drove straight to the clinic and demanded, in a very kind Terri-like way, to see his GP immediately. I was still unaware of any of this....

The News

Vienna and I were reading a book on the couch when Terri came through the front door. "Hi honey, how was your meeting?" I asked.

"Can we talk upstairs?" he responded. I looked at him a little puzzled, as this was an odd request, but I could see there was a panicked look in his eyes.

I turned on Bubble Guppies and let Vienna know we would be upstairs in the bonus room for a few minutes and if she needed me.

As we walked into the bonus room, memories flashed. We still hadn't sold dad's bed or changed much of the décor. It was only 10 days since he had passed, and we were amid planning his funeral. I sighed, getting caught up in the grief of missing dad, and remembering the moments I had with him in hospice before he took his last breath. Cancer is such a beast, I thought. In such a short time, it just ate away at him, and we watched him degrade into unexpressive skin and bones.

Without realizing it, I had stopped in the doorway and was caught up in the painful memories.

"Come and sit with me," Terri said. His words snapped me out of my daze, and I gave him a puzzled look as I had never heard that tone in his voice. That tone—of pain, desperation and complete and utter sadness.

He told me the story of what had happened that morning, and how he had raced to see Dr. Wirasinghe.

The next words out of his mouth were something I never, not in a million years, expected to hear.

"I have Stage IV Pancreatic Cancer."

"Pardon me?" I looked at him in utter disbelief.

When he repeated the words, I started to tremble. I looked at him, seeing tears spring up in the corner of his eyes. He said it again, "Stage IV Pancreatic Cancer."

I am not sure whether it was seconds, minutes, or what felt like a lifetime, but we cried and embraced each other. As I tried to understand what had just happened, Terri explained that the mild indigestion was more than that and the CT showed spots, presumed to be tumors, in his pancreas, lymph nodes, stomach, and many more in his liver.

Once the tears stopped, I took a deep breath, and something snapped inside me. Not in an angry way, not in a defeated way, but in a, "There is no way I am going to lose this amazing man I married," way. He was my husband, the most amazing father to our children, and inherently the most incredible human being I have ever had the privilege of knowing.

I stood, pulled him up to stand with me, took his hands and looked him straight in the eyes.

"This is not happening," I said calmly. "It isn't. You are my husband, and now you are also my project. I will not take anything less than an A++. So... buckle up because we are going to figure this out."

I am not sure he believed me in that moment but as we sit here two and a half years later and he is bordering on cancer free, he knows I was right. There was no giving up, no underestimating and nothing but trust that my man, my hero was going to be around for many, many more years to come.

We were going to expect an unreasonable remission. We were going to think it, create it and manifest it. The only thing I knew for certain was that Terri Mah was going to beat it. The odds were stacked unfavorably, but somewhere deep inside I knew we could do it. He was going to be a survivor.

We share this story as our journey and a testament to faith in God, the Source, the Universe (all interchangeable to me). The importance of trusting instincts, the capability of love and the power of the subconscious mind. There is no one size fits all recipe- but here is our story and we hope it inspires you.

Do you ever wonder if life may throw you the biggest curve balls precisely to help mold you into the person that you were truly meant to be?

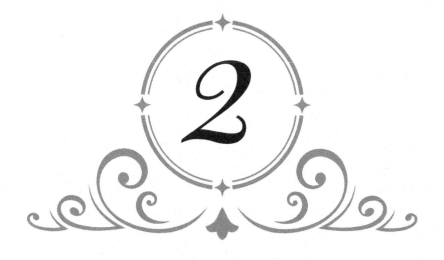

Chapter

A SINKING SHIP—DON'T READ STATISTICS

In the days that followed Terri's diagnosis, life was like a dream. How could this be happening? The thought ran through our minds like a broken record.

We did not tell our children for a long period of time, as we did not want to frighten them. Honestly, how much are little kids supposed to handle? Only two weeks before they had offered kisses and hugs to my dad, their Opa, who was unresponsive on his death bed. Of course, they knew that his demise was due to the *Big C* as well, so we did not want to instill any more fear in them. Years earlier they had also said goodbye to my wonderful mother. Vienna never had the opportunity to get to know her, as she passed away when Vienna was a baby, but we do our best to keep her memory alive in their hearts. Even the move had been traumatic for the kids, and although we were happily settled in Calgary by this point, there had been hardship in the move leaving what they knew as familiar.

As we shared the news with family members and friends, people offered their condolences and looked at us with *that* look. You know, the one that says, "Well you had a good run.... You can't beat this one."

We did our best not to let those looks or sad eyes affect us. Terri, albeit fearful, rose like a Phoenix out of the ashes and refused to believe this would be the end. It was the most powerful human characteristic I have witnessed firsthand.

It is the moments of fear that we face when the soul can triumph!

The first of the appointments began—the biopsy and scopes. Although, these were not our focus. They all went as expected. We sat in the doctor's office, and they told us ever so kindly that they were *so sorry*, that they weren't sure how much time we would have, and that we should meet with the oncologist as soon as possible.

In all honesty, I have such great respect for the medical staff in Canada. At least the ones we have had exposure to. Can you imagine day in and day out delivering heart breaking, life ending news to patients, and trying to support their family and friends? I ask you to consider seeing their job through their eyes as well—

the disappointment they are expected to deliver with positive compassion every single day.

That aside, we were awaiting the biopsy results before meeting with our oncologist. I did not know much at this point, nor did I have direction except on the true power of intuition, but what I did know is this....

Whatever you are facing, whatever you have been told by physicians, do not go home and study statistics. It is like a sinking ship; you will find results offering hopelessness that will make you feel your future is bleak. And yes, it is the reality for many, my dad is a prime example. We were relocating cities in June 2016, and the day they started packing our house was the day that I took my dad to emergency because he wasn't doing well. Pale, lethargic, and less than 100 pounds on a six-foot frame, he was weak and fragile. That very day he was diagnosed with Stage IV Lung Cancer. There were many meetings with doctors and oncologists following—but the point is this.... a few weeks later when the details of dad's diagnosis were confirmed, they gave him an expected nine months to live. How did they determine that number? From analyzing statistics of all those who had passed before with the same condition, they formed a conclusion. Guess what? Would you like to know how long dad lived before he passed? Nine months almost to the day.

Let go of any timeline you have been given. Truly, you must dig deep and believe in your heart that you are not a timeline, nor a statistic—you are you. You are a child born of God with the innate ability to heal your body on a physical, emotional, mental and spiritual level.

Imagine this—you are on a sinking ship, and there is a raft nearby promising a safe passage to land. However, the only way to get to the raft is to make it through the ravaging storm of doubts, the rampant thoughts that say you cannot survive this. Don't let those take root! Face the storm head on. Buckle up, swim through the belief systems, societal influences, and statistics to know that you are capable of more. Survive—you can survive! Whatever you are told, whatever the diagnosis may be, it does not have to be your fate unless you allow it.

I encourage you to read this book and do whatever it takes. I was not equipped with this level of knowledge when my dad went through cancer. Truthfully, it must come from the individual on their own. You can guide. You can empower. You can suggest— but if that deep innate desperation for healing and growth is not there, you cannot fill the gap.

However, you can help. You can teach. If you are reading this book as a caregiver for another, pray for peace, pray for knowledge to help guide, pray that the person you are caring for will attach to the idea that there is so much more beyond the physical level. Pray that life can be changed, no matter what the diagnosis, and that the individual battling does not have to go down with the sinking ship. Understand that they are so much more than a number on a piece of paper. You have the power to change them.

Rather than listening to statistics that say they can take us down, wouldn't the world be an entirely different place if we all viewed our challenges as opportunities to learn and grow?

————————◆————————

Oncology Appointment #1

The *doom day* of oncology appointment #1 arrived. Our good friends—John Kilfoil and Kathryn Wentworth were both physicians and had been very supportive guiding us through the process of trying to understand what we were facing in terms of clinical perspectives. John was kind enough to accompany us to this first oncology appointment to help us process the traumatizing news that we knew was coming our way.

As we sat in the waiting room, I shook impulsively. Trying to be strong for Terri, I did my best to hold my composure. It was so difficult to try and stop the flashbacks of attending these meetings with my father only months earlier. It was almost too much to bear. They haunted my mind. I thrust them away so I could focus on the situation I now faced.

Dr. Scot Dowden shook our hands and sat down with us. It is amazing how much of this journey I remember, yet I recall only a few of his first words. It resembled something like apologizing for the situation we were in, and tactfully trying to provide a ray of hope. We appreciated his kindness and professionalism.

We braced ourselves as we reviewed the first CT Scan. Twenty-four tumors: one in the pancreas, two in the lymph nodes, one in the stomach, and twenty in the liver. CT Scan #1.

The CT results he read (summarized) were as follows:

May 2017

Semi-Urgent Findings: New or unexpected findings that could result in mortality or significant morbidity if not appropriately treated urgently.
Impressions:

1. *Today's CT imaging study confirms the sonographic suspicion of multiple hepatic metastases. More than 20 hypoattenuating lesions are present. Widespread hepatic metastases are the differential diagnosis of exclusion.*

2. *Ill-defined abnormality in the body of the pancreas is extremely concerning for a primary pancreatic adenocarcinoma. Regional lymph nodes are concerning for regional nodal disease. No definite evidence of vascular invasion.*

3. *Multiple peritoneal deposits are worrisome for the presence of peritoneal carcinomatosis.*

Based on the constellation of findings, a primary pancreatic adenocarcinoma with regional nodal metastases, multiple hepatic metastases and peritoneal carcinomatosis with malignant ascites is thought most likely.

"Are you kidding me?" I breathed deeply, again trying to maintain composure.

The tears started flowing and I squeezed Terri's hand to the point of cutting off his circulation. The thoughts flowed—this cannot be happening, this is my man, this is the father to my children.

Although Terri held strong at that moment, I could only imagine the thoughts in his mind. How difficult it must have been to tame the thoughts of impending death.

Realistically, we have all heard about Pancreatic Cancer before. Stage IV. The worst one; the death sentence! No one survives. We have all heard stories, have had loved ones or read about celebrities who were unable to conquer it. Why would Terri be different? I shook my head to dislodge the thought from my mind.

As I reeled back to focusing on the current conversation, and listened to what our doctor was saying, I appreciated how easy it is for others to lose hope. I do not mean that negatively, but rather in a kind and loving way. Our oncologist was being genuine, charismatic, and honestly trying to provide us with the most hope that he could.

What would that resemble though? What did that look like? In the eyes of *the box of Pancreatic Cancer* and all the treatment options available, it all boiled down to chemotherapy. Chemo, chemo and more chemo.

I believe the more precise wording from Dr. Dowden was that he could provide chemo every Monday for Terri, with one Monday off a month. It was genuinely the best that he could offer, and he chose the type of chemo that would be likely to cause the least number of symptoms. He explained that Terri was in the *lucky* group who were quite asymptomatic, and that with continuous chemo he would do his best to keep Terri around for as long as he could. To date, his best success had been a woman who had lived for 5 years after diagnosis.

I respected Dr. Dowden's composure and how he spoke with us. He did not give Terri a timeline or attempt to guesstimate how many months he had to live—even though with the amount of tumors Terri had and to how many locations they had spread, months looked like the case. Simply put, *x* number of months was not an option for me and nor was it for Terri.

I see how people can get overwhelmed with a diagnosis, but Dr. Dowden was so kind, and he provided us with the best information he could. We left thinking that it was a good meeting. That possibly his prognosis was the best hope Terri was going to have…. A few months to a few years.

If we had let that information settle in a little too far—and take root in our subconscious, we would be having an entirely different conversation today.

Have you heard of the iceberg analogy? I didn't know how accurate this was yet, but we have all been taught this in academics in one way or another. Our mind is like an iceberg. Our conscious mind is the tip of the iceberg that we see, only five percent of our mind, leaving our subconscious mind to compose the ninety-five percent that is not seen.

What lives in that subconscious part of our mind and why is it important?

Everything funnels through our subconscious mind and then continues with downward causation to the physical. So, to get to the root cause of our physical issues, such as cancer, we need to go back into the subconscious and understand why it is truly occurring.

Why is it that a principal that has been taught to us all, that seems so simple may seem so foreign when it comes to treating physical pain and illness? The power of the mind can unlock true healing potential.

When the shock of the news wore off, I got to work. I knew there had to be new ways, ideas, treatment options with potential. I wasn't sure. All I knew was that I signed up for at least fifty years of marriage, not ten. Terri Mah was not going anywhere, and together we were going to accomplish the impossible. Without question, I love that man. He lights up a room, and that bright light of his had some work to do to shine the cancer right out of him.

Words of Wisdom

Sylvia Muiznieks is an Advanced BodyTalk Practitioner and instructor. Her talents as both an instructor and practitioner are renowned, and it has been an incredible pleasure training under her guidance. Her words of wisdom guided much of our path in healing, and she shared the most profound explanation of our soul and our light:

Our soul is like a lightbulb shining brightly but is covered with layers of paint—representing the scars of belief systems, memories, traumas and stress—so that the light of who we are can't be seen.

I can only imagine how powerful and synchronized with destiny we can become as we uncover the layers to slowly scratch those blemishes away.

There is nothing that we can't accomplish—including beating Stage IV Pancreatic Cancer. This man of mine is living proof.

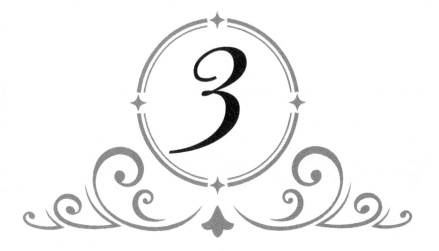

Chapter

DAD'S GREATEST GIFT

My dad was my greatest friend. He was the kind of gentleman who always had a smile on his face and forever wanted to help. Revered by many, he would give the shirt off his back and be there in a split second if you were in a pinch.

"Dad, would you be able to pick up the kids from preschool today?" I would call and ask him. "Absolutely, I will be right there," he would respond with loving kindness.

"Dad, any chance you could babysit Friday night? Terri and I would like to go out to a movie." His response never ceased to amaze me. "Thank you for the opportunity," he would say, and I could hear his smile through the phone.

When we lived in Saskatoon, we used to have dates with him Wednesdays. That day was Terri's Men's Golf Night, and he always looked forward to it. Dad would whip around in his bright blue Honda Civic after work (like he was a race car driver) and pop out ever so eagerly. The kids would open the door for him as he arrived and start waving from the front entrance. "Opa is here mom, Opa is here!"

We would walk over to nearby restaurants, and let the kids ride their bikes. We would chit chat over dinner, talking about the day and how his business was going. We all enjoyed our time together so much. There are so many pictures of those Wednesday dates, with ketchup covered faces when the kids were tiny, and playground antics on the way home afterwards.

When dad was diagnosed, and we were relocating to Calgary, we convinced him to move with us. I wanted to take care of him and did not want any distance between us. It was such a blessing that he decided he would come, and it was also incredibly heavy on his heart.

Relocating for dad meant leaving his home of forty years, the home where he and mom had raised my brother and me, a home filled with a lifetime of memories. It also meant leaving his computer consulting business, his true passion, and serving clients only from a distance.

Dad was in and out of the hospital over the summer, and we rallied to pack his house up and put it on the market. We thought it would be less painful (to some extent) if we could go through items as proficiently as possible while he was in hospital. It was overwhelming—we had our whole house to pack up and move, so we had to be selective in how many of his possessions could accompany us.

This was one of my first lessons about worldly possessions. Filing through papers now, I often wonder why we hang on to so much? In the end, those possessions do not provide joy, rather they only clutter our hearts and minds.

Before dad moved to Calgary, they did multiple doses of radiation. The tumor in his lungs was nine by twelve centimeters and had eaten through his ribs and around into his back. Even with that successful bout of radiation, dad still lived the exact amount of time he had been *given* by the professional medical teams that diagnosed him.

This book is not intended to focus on my dad, but it is important to inspire the question of *why* challenges and obstacles happen in our lives.

Throughout the following months of dad living with us, we had some great times. The kids loved having him in the house, and he was so thrilled to come to every hockey game, soccer game, gymnastics class—whatever he could view. It was so very special. Even when he had to haul his oxygen tank and things were becoming more difficult, he would still attend.

At the end of March, dad went into palliative care in the hospital. A few weeks later, he was perking up and I thought he would come home again. I was so optimistic. In retrospect, I see now it had to happen this way. How would we have possibly handled two Stage IV Cancer patients in our house at the same time?

At that time, I didn't understand though, and it was so painful to watch him slowly just fade away. He moved into hospice a month later and was there for five days before he passed away.

The morning they were moving him from the hospital, they had forgotten to give him his pain medication. Although he was in excruciating pain because of it, it was also a blessing. He had a lucid moment, and as I held his hand, he looked at me and thanked me repeatedly for everything I had done for him, for being his daughter, and for all the love we shared. I wept as I heard the love in his voice, and knew I was also releasing the pain of knowing he was not going to be with us much longer. We were always affectionate with each other and I had heard these kind words before, but it is amazing how much more they can mean when someone is on their death bed. If we took people's kind words to heart every day, imagine how much brighter a place the world would be.

When we knew dad had only hours left, I packed a bag to stay with him at hospice. During his last thirty hours he became completely unresponsive and was unable to even move his eyebrows as he had before. I kept reassuring him to let him know I was there. As the hours passed, I felt a sense of urgency. I needed to do something, help in some way with the transition, so dad could go as peacefully as possible. I wanted to let him know just how much we loved him.

In those tearful and painful moments, watching him lie in bed, I saw the soul of my dad emerging. Metaphorically, I could feel a beautiful white light rising while his body faded. There was no movement left in his limbs, and under each prominent bone was a small pillow to caress the area. Kind volunteers had sewn these pillows with love, and some were heart shaped. They protected his elbows, hips and knees from more intense pain than he was already experiencing.

My heart and soul knew I could be strong enough to be there for my dad to support him, but I did not want to witness him take his last breath. For some reason, that would just be much more than I could bear.

I went for a walk, thinking the fresh air would clear my head. I prayed to God for a peaceful passing and trusted in advance how happy dad would be in heaven. Honestly, I was also giving dad time to know I was there but maybe just far enough away for him to slip away.

When I returned, I was struck with a sense of clarity—knowing exactly what I needed to do. Even though I was afraid of hurting him, I crawled into bed and lay beside him. A nurse covered me with a blanket while I wept and wept. I took my phone out of my pocket and queued up "Amazing Grace."

"Dad," I said. "I know this is just what you need. It's your favorite song. Please know that I will always love you and I will take care of everything. I promise. It is safe for you to go now."

The most incredible thing happened, as soon as he heard the music of his most endearing song, he raised his eyebrows and tried to smile. He had made no movement in the past thirteen hours and I knew God had given me the strength to provide him just what he needed.

I played "Amazing Grace" repeatedly. I played it with lyrics, with his favorite Scottish Bagpipes, and I reminded him constantly how much I loved him.

When the exhaustion overtook me, I told him one more time that he was so special, and I thanked him, for being the best dad in the world. I explained that I was quite scared of hurting him and I was going to lie in the recliner next to him. After being awake for over thirty hours with him, I was sound asleep in seconds.

Less than ten minutes later, the charge nurse woke me and let me know that dad had passed away. He had gone so peacefully.

This was an epic situation where I chose to stay tuned in to God and the Universe and trust my instincts. It was my moment with dad, and it was a gift that I was given to have that time with him. I trusted the insight to help make his final moments so special and everlasting. Those moments are forever bound on my heart.

The Underlying Meaning

This is not a book about my father, but this is an important lesson. When you open yourself up to the true meaning of why things happen, it will bring peace to your heart and understanding.

Even though I miss him dearly every day, I know and trust that dad—both as a father and friend, gave me the most honouring and special gift he could. He gave me the gift of keeping my husband.

He took me through the journey of cancer to realize the limitations that existed, how deep we must dig, and how incredibly strong willed and full of true faith we must be to overcome something intended to take us down.

The strength is not only needed from the patient themselves, but for a caregiver as well. We endure the experience in such a different way. My desperation, my hope, and my research led me to all the options I needed to save Terri's life. Terri had the incredibly difficult task of remaining optimistic, enduring treatments and changing— but together we did it.
My dad's greatest gift was to give me many more years of marriage, family and a divine sense of gratitude. Thank you, dad. There will never be words large enough to express my appreciation.

Next time there is doubt in your heart as to how to heal, solve a problem, or rebuild relationships—do as I did here. Dig deep to understand and look at the big picture. Look for signs. Make lemonade out of lemons. Hold strong and fast.

Don't give up—we all have incredible destinies we can realize. But we must get out of our own way to listen, find and achieve them.

Imagine if we all tried to find the silver lining in every situation. Imagine the possibilities that could unfold.

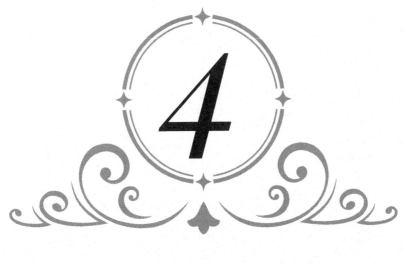

Chapter

THE SCIENCE OF THE SUBCONSCIOUS MIND

As the days unfolded, I spent them smiling and entertaining my children, and nights searching in desperation for answers (still refusing to read statistics). Researching clinics world-wide. Once I started looking, there were infinite options, it was just a matter of narrowing it down and finding the right clinic for us.

In the meantime, as the search went on, we did what else we could. Terri started drinking a lot of carrot juice, and I mean a lot. We are lucky he didn't turn orange! He started taking CBD oil, which also has numerous testimonials as to the impact it has had on cancer.

I knew in my heart that this would be the beginning of energy healing in our lives. I had a friend of many years who was a BodyTalk Practitioner, and immediately when I spoke to her, I asked her to start doing three BodyTalk sessions a week on Terri. I also knew that I needed to learn BodyTalk, how it worked and the true impact it could have on health and happiness.

I recall it being a Tuesday that I spoke to her, and by no coincidence there was a Mindscape class (a class within the BodyTalk system) being taught the weekend following. I packed up my bags and drove back to Saskatoon to take the class. I didn't like the thought of leaving Terri at this time, but I knew in my heart that what I would be learning would well be worth the time away. Little did I know just how much of an impact it would have on our entire wellbeing.

———————————————◆————————————————

Keesje

On a side note, we were really struggling with having my dad's dog with us. We loved her very much, but it was hard for her since dad had passed away, and I prayed for a sign as to what we should do with her. She was getting quite old and was not used to having so many people around. Our kids are social so on any given day there were a handful of kids running up and down the stairs.

Then it happened—our kind neighbour had brought over a healthy smoothie for Terri, and Keesje bit her son right on the lip. In her kindness, she was using it as an educational moment for her son on how to approach dogs, but for me I knew that was the straw that broke the camel's back. Sad as I was, Keesje could no longer live with us.

It was no coincidence this happened, and only a few days later I was driving to Saskatoon. My brother was kind enough to have Keesje live with him on his acreage and she was very happy there.

When you start trying to understand occurrences and why they happen, your perspective begins to shift, and new realizations begin to unfold.

As Abraham Hicks describes in the following quote, we had aligned to the destiny of Keesje needing a new home.

Anything that's happening right now is old news. Because the vibration flowed a long time ago. And it took time for it to manifest into something that is tangible. But even when it's happening right now, in terms of what you're hearing, or seeing, or so forth, it's old news. Because the new stuff is in this vibrational reality. So, if you could, just for a little while—we know it's not easy, especially under extreme conditions—if you could notice less of what is, and talk more about what you desire, on that subject and all others, you will become, every day more, a vibrational match to your own preferences. And anything that does not match that preference will vibrate out of your experience.

———————————◆———————————

Power of the Mind

Now, this is where I may lose some of you, or you may think, "Is she just making this up?"; "Do these methods really work?" I implore you to continue reading. My very healthy and whole husband is living proof that they certainly can bring success.

The most interesting fact is that I had been exposed to BodyTalk a few years before. My first session stirred up so many emotions; it took a good month of processing. Following that though, I started having more regular sessions, some on my kids, and noticed positive changes in how I was feeling. Terri always said he believed in the power of the mind, but that it was too nonspecific for him. He was not willing to explore further, as it was out of his comfort zone. That is, until he was diagnosed and forced to reconsider.

Trying to look at the cosmic way of how events play out, if I had not had exposure over the years, I would not have been so keen for my friend to start so many sessions on Terri.

———————————◆———————————

The BodyMind Connection

In Debbie Shapiro's *The BodyMind Workbook,* she introduces the concept that the body and mind co-exist, which is also the foundation for all BodyTalk and MindScape work. A key passage reads as follows:

To understand the bodymind connection, we first have to recognize that the mind and body are one. Generally, we regard the body as something we carry about with us (often somewhat reluctantly), something that is easily damaged, that needs exercise, regular food and water, a certain amount of sleep and occasional check-ups. The body becomes a great nuisance when it is damaged, so then we take it to a doctor in the belief that he or she will be able to mend it, and the quicker the better. Something is broken, so we go to get it fixed- as if this 'something' is an inanimate object, devoid of intelligence. When the body is functioning well, we are happy, we feel alive and energetic. When it is not, we soon become irritated, frustrated, depressed, and full of self-pity.

The view of the body is sadly limited. It denies the complexity of the energies that make up our entire being, energies that are constantly communicating and flowing between each other; between our thoughts, feelings, and the physical maintenance of our various parts. There is no separation between what is happening in our minds and what is happening in our bodies; relatively we do not exist separate to the body in which we have our existence. Consider how in the English language we think of someone with great presence as a 'somebody,' while a person with little significance is a 'nobody.' Our bodies are us; our state of being is a direct result of the communication between the numerous different aspects of our existence. To say, 'I have hurt my

*arm,' is to say that 'a hurt inside of me is manifesting in my arm.'
What the hurt in the arm is expressing is not different from verbal
expressions of anger or confusion. To say there is a difference is to
ignore the essential unity of the whole being. To treat only the arm
is to disregard the source of the pain that the arm is manifesting.
Denying this bodymind relationship is ignoring the opportunity
that the body gives us to look at, accept and resolve our inner
pain.[1]*

This bodymind connection opens the door to possibilities. You
can absolutely consider yourself the most positive person, and
the biggest of dreamers. But what if there is more? What if
cracking through the barriers of our limited conscious minds opens
unlimited possibilities?

As you stretch past the capabilities of the known conscious mind,
into the breaming and limitless powers of the subconscious mind,
not only do we connect deeper with God and the Universe, but
we bring into our awareness the truth that we can accomplish
anything.

Let that sink in. We can accomplish anything! We are created
with the innate wisdom and power to heal ourselves, manifest
beautiful destinies, and transform our lives.

How do we do it? Thinking back to the iceberg analogy, our
conscious mind makes up roughly five percent of our mind,
and our subconscious mind makes up ninety-five percent. From
reading that fact alone, where do you think you can affect the
most change?

When we are born, we are an entirely subconscious being. As we
grow and form our identities, we start forming habits, patterns
and belief systems. By the age of six or seven we have formed so
many of our belief systems that they inherently govern our day
to day activities and thought processes. As Dr. Bruce H. Lipton is
quoted saying:

*Our thoughts are mainly controlled by our subconscious, which
is largely formed before the age of 6, and you cannot change to*

---

[1]Debbie Shapiro, *The BodyMind Workbook, Exploring how the Mind and The Body Work
Together* (Great Britain: Element Books Limited, 1990), 1-2

subconscious mind by just thinking about it... The subconscious mind is like a tape player. Until you change the tape, it will not change.

Sylvia has always reminded me that it all comes down to one simple principle. "It all comes down to consciousness," she would say with a smile. Her presence in the classroom was so calming and welcoming. She would explain how the bodymind is all connected, and that to achieve healing we need to break our attachments to belief systems that are buried within our subconscious (the bottom of the iceberg). It was incredible that each time she would teach an Advanced Class, the material and techniques would vary, but always circled back to this principle.

Let's look at an example: your ten-year-old child is adamant that she does not like tomatoes. She refuses to eat them—in salad, in spaghetti sauce, in any way, shape or form. Where did that come from? Why do they have such a strong aversion to tomatoes? When you ask the question, you receive the response, "I don't know, mom…. I just don't like them."

When you look at this in a broader prospective, and you understand that your subconscious mind is governing and controlling that ninety-five percent of our lives, we need to look deeper.

Perhaps the first time that you fed your child tomatoes, it was a rainy Sunday. Your husband had been called into work that afternoon, and you were tired and overwhelmed. Secretly, you had been hoping to have some help with housework that day, and to have a break from the toddler who was wonderful but ever so demanding. Nonetheless, you appreciated the importance of his meeting, and tried not to hold it against him. However, as you were making spaghetti for supper, you felt the anger brewing. You took a deep breath and reminded yourself not to start a fight. Supper was on the table warm and delicious, and you took the extra effort to bake a fresh loaf of bread with the meal. As he walked in the door, he was so annoyed that it had been raining and, as a result, the bottom of his pants and shoes were soaked. It was an utter downpour, and his mood reflected the state of the weather outside.

Well, that was it. "How could he possibly be grumpy about stupid rain?" you thought. I am the one who has been slaving away and managing a toddler, and I even went to the extra effort of making this wonderful meal.

You take another deep breath and serve up dinner. Taking tiny bites, your toddler looking at you with expectant eyes. You ask your husband how his day was. Boom! The anger flows out, "Didn't you see I ruined my pants?"; "Do you think I like working Sundays?".... And the complaints go on and on.

Deep breaths are no longer working, and you fight back. "I would gladly trade you days for a break," is the first sentence out of your mouth. Words go back and forth, escalating into yelling, and soon a plate is slammed onto the table. It breaks, and warm spaghetti sauce oozes down the side of the table.

Tears well up in your toddler's eyes. As dad storms away mad, and you run to the kitchen to get a cloth to clean the spaghetti sauce and broken dish, your toddler is left sitting alone strapped in their highchair at the dining room table.

Eating what? Spaghetti sauce. Made of what? Tomatoes. Just like that—his subconscious mind has taken a snapshot of that entire situation, like a perfect photo. Yelling parents, broken plates, messy table, and tomatoes.

Why does your ten-year-old refuse to eat tomatoes? Because as a toddler, from that experience alone, it is possible she locked in her subconscious mind that tomatoes are yucky, scary, dangerous and invoke feelings of fear on a deep level that they are not even aware of. Consciously, they have no recollection of this event, and really cannot explain why they do not like tomatoes; although subconsciously, that event created a belief system that tomatoes were not safe.

Wow! This is the truth of how diving into your subconscious can truly unlock things we are not even aware of. This is the understanding that every physical issue—whether it be an allergy, an illness, arthritis, cancer, auto-immune disorder comes from the mind. Like a trickle-down effect, if we are not dealing with events or occurrences that have framed themselves into our subconscious mind, they then work their way through the bodymind complex in order to get our attention and be addressed. When an unresolved emotion/event is not addressed within our bodymind complex, it has a downward causation. If it is continually unaddressed, it flows downward until it gets our attention with physical symptoms.

Chocolate Trauma

Similar to the above story, and sharing a vulnerable personal example, I was allergic to chocolate. I had no idea where this allergy came from or what triggered it. If I ate chocolate of any kind, I would have a headache and then would vomit. It was an odd reaction to a food, but that is what happened, and it certainly was not enjoyable.
The odd thing was that I had fond memories of days when my brother and I would roll around in the puddles in front of our house and become freezing cold. Why would we do such a silly thing? Because the reaction on my dad's face, when we would ring the front doorbell in such a state, was one of pure enjoyment and happy disposition. What would our reward be? A nice hot cup of cocoa to warm us up. At that point, the chocolate caused my physical body no harm.

So, where did this allergy come from? If I had those memories, how did it now make sense that every time I ate or drank chocolate, I would be ill?

It took a lot of energetic work, and hundreds of BodyTalk sessions for the truth to emerge.

I was a figure skater when I was young. I was passionate about skating, and I loved being at the rink. It was only a block from our house in the small town we lived in, and I would walk over after school on my own for my lessons. My mom would always pack me thermoses of hot milk and honey for the journey and for in between lessons. It was a metal rink, literally a tin can, with real ice, and it was cold. Like warm your toes in your mittens cry and between lessons cold.

For years, I wondered why I suddenly lost my passion for skating. I was unable to do jumps of any kind and was also very uncomfortable at the rink. The old caretaker had left, and I would often babysit the kids of the new caretaker. I often felt hesitant around that caretaker for no apparent reason, and I really was not sure why.

I'll fill in the blanks for you. The old caretaker did not retire or disappear. He went to jail. He was charged with many counts of sexual assault of children that took skating lessons in our rink. I always wondered why I was one of the few lucky ones that was not assaulted?

I always knew deep down that I was not one of the lucky ones, but I did not remember any abusive events, so in my adolescence I did not spend a lot of time focusing on it. I knew that there must be a reason why I stopped figure skating as a teen, and why I felt so uncomfortable at the rink.

Years later, when a family member who is very in tune with consciousness wanted to consult with me about *dissociative state,* I knew exactly what was going to come up. In a way, I was appreciative. Appreciative that through my younger years I did not need to be in the media, face this trauma or involve my parents. I had not been one of the lucky ones. I was sexually assaulted by the caretaker of the rink. I had blocked it out for years, but only in my conscious mind. It was always very much alive in my subconscious mind. How did it dictate that it needed my attention—at some point and in some way?

Can you guess what the caretaker used to feed us? Chocolate bars. He used to invite us into *his room* and welcome us onto his lap. He would feed us chocolate bars as a comfort.

So, my conscious mind was not ready to process this for many years but needed to make it known to my physical body that it was on the radar to be figured out. How did it do that? My *allergy* to chocolate.

After much deep work in my subconscious mind, not only am I over this event, but I can also eat chocolate. By the bits, by the scoopful, by the handful, by the truck load if I choose.

The *allergy* is gone. I determined the root cause of what placed it there, this horrible childhood molestation; and I worked through it all. I am healed from the trauma and memories of that experience on the physical level, because I worked through it on the subconscious level.

This is no different than Terri working through his cancer. The physical symptom of cancer was there, with a root cause in the subconscious mind. By working through the layers of masks, doubts and belief systems in the subconscious mind, not only are you free from the physical pain and discomfort, but you are lighter in all levels of consciousness.

Can you imagine if we all analyzed our physical symptoms as a representation of something deeper going on in our subconscious mind? How much could we possibly heal and help each other? It would be a transformation beyond our wildest imagination.

———————————◆———————————

Journey of Looking Within

Truth be told, you should always trust your intuition. Your gut is always right. It led me to uncovering why I was *allergic* to chocolate. More importantly, it confidently led me to the road Terri, and I should take for his healing.

Let's put this into perspective. This diagnosis, this limited future according to Western Medicine. Yet, here we stand—united and strong. Terri is healthier than he ever has been. Not only have his physical symptoms shifted and dissipated, but our marriage, respect for each other, and how we raise our children is resoundingly different. Not that we are perfect in any manner, but the profound work and effort we put in daily has created big healing.

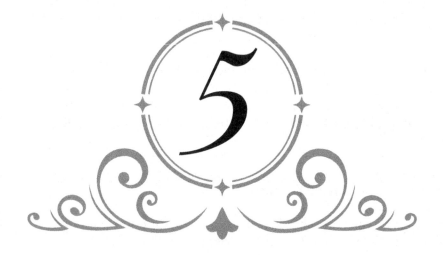

Chapter

MINDSCAPE—A POWERFUL TOOL

Do you know what the biggest factor of Terri's successful healing was? Barre none, it's the fact that whether he meant to or not, by the road I guided him down, it became a journey of looking within. The greatest change comes from our own deep dive into the darkest places and trying to understand what our physical symptoms and life's experiences are trying to teach us. The willingness to be vulnerable and connect with God and the Universe to awaken your potential. What are they trying to awaken us to? In which reality do we want to be living? A happy, healthy, positive one is within our grasp if we are willing to do the work.

As I drove back to Saskatoon, music turned loud and window down the breeze flowing in, I recapped the last year of our lives. I reflected on how we thought that moving to Calgary was such a big deal or remembering when I took my dad to hospital and we received his horrible diagnosis.

None of that paled in comparison to what I was feeling now, or most certainly what Terri was feeling. Strangely enough, I knew he was going to be okay. With dad, I knew we would cherish his last few months, and help him to make a timely transition to heaven. It was a complete and utterly different experience now. In the moments with Terri, I felt the peace and love of God resonating in me and giving me the faith, and strength, to trust Terri was going to survive and thrive. That strength was a blessing. It gave me the ability to have the insight to focus my research and thoughts towards decisions resulting in an incredible health outcome. We needed to step outside of the box. Actually—we needed to do so much more than step outside of the box. More accurately put, we needed to allow and accept the awareness and realization that the box does not exist. It cannot hold you back because the only box that exists governs the limitations of your mind that you choose to accept.

When I arrived for day one of MindScape class, I wondered what I was getting myself into. It seemed so foreign to me, but I knew with certainty that my mind needed to expand, my earth needed to be shattered, and my husband needed to be saved. He was going to be that one—the man who changes protocol, opens eyes, warms hearts and becomes a picture of perfect health.

Imagine if we all took the time to look past the horrible diagnosis, the failing marriage or the anxiety plaguing us, to break down the walls and realize that the box does not exist. What possibilities lie there, in the vast and untouched expanse of our subconscious minds and the quantum realm? What can we transform? The more apt question—what can't we not transform? The answer is nothing. Absolutely nothing is impossible, unreachable or incurable. Absolutely nothing.

———————————————◆————————————————

What is MindScape?

The definition of MindScape on the International BodyTalk Association Website reads as follows:

MindScape offers a window into the powerful insights of your right-brain creative mind.

Its foundations are around tapping into and utilizing the capabilities of our subconscious mind, that ninety-five percent that governs much of our lives without us even thinking about it.

My favorite quote comes from Albert Einstein:

You cannot fix a problem in the same level of consciousness that created it.

What does that mean? Regardless if we are a positive thinker, a happy go lucky soul, unless we get to the root programming of the subconscious mind, it is much more difficult and much more unlikely that we are going to affect great change in our lives—in any physical, mental, or emotional capacity.

MindScape is a class within the BodyTalk system, created by Dr. John Veltheim. It provides a tool to easily and quickly access your subconscious mind. Once there, you can fully realize that all information is accessible, and all potential is unlimited.

Sylvia's principles of teaching MindScape and training instructors rely on tapping into the immense opportunities for growth, healing and understanding that lies within the subconscious.

There are so many incredible tools that resonate differently with everyone. I believe that every individual should delve into working with their subconscious mind and to investigate which modalities resonate with them. The life-changing events that make your jaw drop do not always occur after going into MindScape just once or accessing your subconscious in another way. It comes with a daily commitment, and time. Like exercise or healthy eating, our physical body takes time to respond and adjust to the changes implemented.

The first time I took the class in Saskatoon was with instructor Kristin Pierce. She herself had used the power of the mind to overcome her own cancer journey; she had an incredible energy to share. She has utilized her MindScape skills to overcome obstacles, manifest a destiny she desired, and she has become a successful children's author. She is an inspiration as to how MindScape can transform your life.

As we sat in the classroom, she explained how we may feel some resistance. That our protective ego, or left brain, is literally wondering what we are trying to accomplish. As Dr. Joe Dispenza says:

95% of who we are by the time we're thirty-five years old is a memorized set of behaviors, emotional reactions, unconscious habits, hardwired attitudes, beliefs and perceptions that function like a computer program.

In other words, when we are brave enough to delve in, and look beyond the walls we have created, we will shake things up. It takes time, effort and persistence for our ego to step out of the way and let us get past our own barriers of resistance.

Kristin coined the phrase *Nice Kitty* for us to speak to our egos during the MindScape exercise if the resistance was too strong. What does that feel like? We experience it every day in life; have you ever had a wonderful inspiring daydream take you away to a magical place just when you catch yourself saying, "That's not possible," or "You do not have the skills to accomplish that?" Acknowledging that our ego is trying to protect us in these situations allows us to move past it and trust that our instincts may just be showing us a new way to our inspired true destiny.

Can you imagine if we all listened to our inner voices? The ones that say, "Yes, be brave and apply for that amazing career," or "Go for it—write a book," or in this case more aptly, "You can beat Stage IV Pancreatic Cancer." We all have it within us to become what we can only imagine in our wildest dreams.

What if we all took a moment when the resistance popped up to thank ourselves, and our ego for trying to protect us? Then we could shift gears and embark on a new and unmarked path. That we are going to take the opportunity and carve out a new destiny. That we are going to work through and change our deeply programmed life and manifest new and magnificent outcomes.

How would the world look if we all chose this path? We can only dream that as more and more of us begin on the journey of deep change, the better our own futures and collective destiny will be.

———————————◆◆———————————

Eyes Wide Open

When I completed MindScape, mind blown and eyes wide open, I flew home ready to attempt to explain to Terri what I had experienced. Not only was I keen to share with him the tools I learned but also to show how connected we all are.

Simply put, when you are in MindScape, in your subconscious mind, you are connected to the infinite field of possibilities. This does not just include outcomes, but also the ability to connect with people.

Based on Quantum Physics, we are all just energy, comprised of waves and particles, and we are all connected. In MindScape class we learned that we are able to invite another individual into our minds to connect with them, of course the first person I reached out to was Terri. Desperate to try and help him, I felt that I could offer some sort of treatment for him while I was in my subconscious mind.

On the plane ride home, I went into my workshop and I invited Terri in. A workshop is a sacred place you create in your subconscious, an elaborate process you go through in the

MindScape class. It is so fun, and you can create a space that is truly you. When Terri was invited in, at first, he was very perplexed and curious about my space, and then very intrigued. I showed him around with pride and took him into my library. I asked him to see if my book was there, the one I was going to write about him beating this cancer. According to Albert Einstein, time and space are an illusion, so this future book should be accessible now, in the present moment. It was a lofty goal, and I was not sure that a book would reveal itself.

Amazingly, it did. I could not believe it. I became even more certain in that moment that Terri was going to be a survivor. He was going to be a game changer. A healed man offering hope and inspiration to those struggling with cancer around the world.

We were guided in my workshop to Aisle six, book 4B. We held hands as we walked through my library, and I gave Terri more details on how we are all connected. A good friend explained it like this—think of it as cell phones. Imagine if we would have told our grandparents that one day, we would be able to speak with someone on a cell phone across the world without land lines. That would be a shocking revelation. Understandably, some may find it difficult at first to realize that we are all connected. The more we do the work, the more the possibilities abound, and perceptions are blown wide open. It is such an incredible journey.

As we arrived in Aisle six, we scanned the shelves for book 4B. I had no idea what to expect. Being so new to MindScape, I wondered if my ego was possibly playing tricks on me. Trust the process, Kristie Anne. Believe in possibilities.

Nervously I laid my hands on this white hard covered book that had 4B written in red letters on the side. As my fingers touched the cover, pulsing sensations ran through my entire body. I looked at the front cover and it said this:

The Day the Cancer Quit

A True Story of Surviving Stage IV Pancreatic Cancer

Kristie Anne Mah

There it was! In that moment, I was reminded once again that my husband was going to be okay. I received such amazing signs so early in the journey. Clearly God knew I needed those reminders to keep strong and keep my head in the game. He knew I needed the strength to figure out the tumultuous battle that lay ahead.

What would happen if we all approached our days differently? If instead of trying to simply survive, we allowed ourselves to be open to all those little signs and reminders that the Universe and God (to me they are one in the same, but it is entirely personal preference) are showing to us through our intuition, and through external triggers? What different journeys we might all have....

Treatment Lesson 101

After we relished in the fact that my book did in fact exist, we stored it back on the shelf in my library, and I asked Terri to join me in my healing room. It was a sacred space I had created to try and develop some understanding of which treatments were going to benefit Terri.

After all, we stopped reading statistics, but certainly were aware that the odds were stacked against us. No one heard of individuals beating Pancreatic Cancer, let alone Stage IV. You only heard of those that it defeated, and how quickly at that. If Patrick Swayze and Steve Jobs could not beat it, why should I believe that Terri could? They had all the money in the world for treatments. Success is going to come from treating all of Terri, I reminded myself, not just the treatments that consisted of Western Medicine. Those do not get past the conscious mind or physical body. They serve their purpose, but on their own they are not enough. I didn't know yet what was required, but I certainly knew that we needed to address his cancer from a full picture perspective: BodyTalk, MindScape, faith and prayer—looking at the physical, mental, emotional and spiritual combined.

When we were sitting in my healing room, I became emotional that Terri had been given this burden of cancer. I told him that I was going to do my best to get it out of him. I knew I could guide him, but ultimately the work came down to him. His determination. His willingness. I have always been a dreamer, and once I was in MindScape, I enjoyed letting my right brain guide the process, and trusting whatever whimsical, creative, or silly thoughts might enter.

As we held hands sitting on the love seat in my healing room, I took a deep breath and wondered what I could do to destroy the cancer. Lemmings popped into my mind! I'm not sure if you ever played that old school computer game, but it was one of my favorites. There were a group of these little creatures, lemmings, that you would have to lead together collectively to make it through obstacles to complete the level. If you did not have them working together, they would end up walking off a cliff or trapped against a wall, and you would fail a level.

"Why can't my little lemmings work together to destroy Terri's cancer?" I thought. So, that's what I did. I sent little lemmings into my husband's stomach to destroy the cancer. Of course, this was in my workshop in my MindScape, essentially it was my subconscious working on his hologram.

I felt proud of myself and had a little nap on the plane before I landed back in Calgary. Remembering just how new I was at all of this, I was not sure if my work had accomplished anything, but I had attempted to try and help. After going through dad's Stage IV Lung Cancer, that is arguably the most difficult part. You can love, support, drive to appointments, make sandwiches, and change Fentanyl patches, but beyond that I felt helpless. A bystander witnessing a most magnificent person withering away. I refused to be that person again. I had to be able to do something more to help my wonderful husband.

All Connected

When I landed in Calgary, I was embraced by Terri and my kids with open arms. I had only been gone a few days, but it was so good to see them again. Nixon told me about his hockey games, and Vienna asked me if I brought her any presents. "Not on such a short trip, honey—but why don't we watch your favorite show together later," I replied.

The kids were occupied in the back of the truck doing their best to keep up with the lyrics of "Shake it Off," and the strangest thing happened.

"My stomach really hurts," Terri mentioned. "It has not hurt like this ever, not before the diagnosis, through the testing, or even afterwards. It has never hurt like this." He cringed a little and clasped onto his left side, right over top of where his pancreas is located.

"Are you kidding me?" I asked. My heart raced and my cheeks flushed. My mind was processing at what felt like a million miles a minute. "Could it be?" I wondered to myself. "Is there any chance?"

"What do you mean am I kidding you?" Terri looked at me a little shocked. "Is there something I don't know...." he paused and wondered if he should utter the next statement. "Did you do something?" he asked.

I puzzled at how to respond. I had not even had the opportunity to explain to Terri how wonderful the MindScape class had been, and how passionate I felt about it. How it already poured through my blood, and I wanted to shout from the rooftops how everyone should learn this amazing technique and powerful tool.

I took a deep breath and sighed. "What do I have to lose?" I thought. "I might as well tell him...."

"I..."

"Well, I..."

"What are you trying to say to me?" Terri asked, now intrigued as to how I could have possibly contributed to the extra discomfort in his stomach.

"To make a long story short," I started off, "In MindScape they taught us how we are all connected. I invited you into my workshop, drilled little holes in your stomach and sent Lemmings to destroy the cancer." I realized that I was speaking quietly thinking it would somehow lessen the apparent craziness of the story I was telling him.

I swear that he almost drove off the road. "What do you mean?" he asked, perplexed and obviously needing more clarity.

As we continued the drive, I went on to explain the foundations of the course, and how powerful it can be. By the end of the conversation, I could still see the wide-eyed look on Terri's face, but there was one thing that we agreed upon.

He did feel it. No question. The sensations and discomfort were different than they ever had been before, and although it did not yet sit well with our logical minds, we did agree. My treatment on Terri's hologram, in my subconscious mind, was felt by him on a physical level.

Thank you, God, for confirming ever so quickly that we were on the right path, and that You will put amazing opportunities and skills in my wheelhouse to conquer this cancer.

Chapter

DON'T FIGHT YOUR CANCER, LOVE IT

I heard the patter of footsteps coming down the hallway, and I stretched and rolled over. Looking at the clock, and realizing it was already after 8am I sat straight up in bed. I quickly had my two little monkeys on me, one giving me a Nixon-blanket as we called it, and Vienna snuggling right into my armpit.

"Ooooh smelly," she said and giggled. It was a long-standing joke that either my armpit or breath was of some great stench in the morning. I gave her a tickle, and she hopped on top of Nixon for a sandwich cuddle before we started the morning.

I was absolutely amazed at how well I had slept, since I had not been able to stay asleep for more than a couple of hours at a time since Terri was diagnosed. It's mind-blowing when you challenge your brain at a new level, how rewarding it can be, and how it can provide pure rest as well.

Terri hopped out of bed. We made breakfast for the kiddos and off they went. Nixon had school that morning, and since he was in Grade Two, he biked with a couple of buddies. Vienna had gymnastics, so I made a coffee for the road and took her there.

As I sat in gymnastics, my mind began to wander as to how we got here. Ten years married, now in Calgary, wonderful kids, parents already passed, friendships come and gone, and now unequivocally the biggest battle of our life.

I took a deep breath and realized just how strong our foundation was. Terri and I had been through a lot together, and without doubt I knew we were going to succeed at this. Not just make it through but succeed. Beat it, conquer it, and share it with the world. I took a moment to reflect on how my journey with Terri had began...

Strangers at First

It was early in the morning as I sat down in my new office. It was not my dream job by any stretch, but if I wanted to get into the pharmaceutical industry, I knew I needed something strong on my resume. A Fortune 500 company ought to do the trick.

As I was trying to understand the computer program, I heard the ding of the doorbell, and then outrageous laughter. It quickly became clear that whoever was visiting was good buddies with my colleague. They were telling jokes, and I heard this guy ask who took over his job. Deke wandered over and introduced us.

"Taking over his job," I thought to myself. He must be a friend of Deke's. "If he is here all the time, is he just going to be a pain in the butt?" I internally rolled my eyes but stood to be polite.

"Meet Kristie Anne," Deke said kindly. He joked about how I had big shoes to fill, and how I owned a car with a loud muffler but that I seemed to be alright.

"Kristie Anne meet Terri. Terri Mah." I shook his hand and we smiled cordially, never in a million years thinking that, not too far into the future, he would be the love of my life.

———————————◆———————————

Which Clinic to Choose?

In the afternoon, things became a little emotional again. We were staying very strong for the most part, but when researching new and innovative ways to treat pancreatic cancer, without doubt I stumbled across statistics. We had made a pledge not to read the statistics as they were entirely doom and gloom. We knew that if we let a thought grab hold in our mind, and we remind ourselves of it every day, it takes root in our subconscious, and eventually plays out in our reality because we believe it so deeply.

Imagine if we all took the time to acknowledge the negative or damaging thoughts that entered our minds, thanked them for coming into our awareness, and then instructed them to leave, replacing them with entirely positive and motivating thoughts? We could manifest destinies of health, wholeness and dreams fulfillment. Who says that a dream cannot come true? Only our words create our barriers. I kept reminding myself that my dream, of all dreams, was to help cure my husband's Stage IV Cancer. I would somehow, someway, through the grace of God find the path of treatments he needed. I had no doubt Terri was strong enough to do the work, and together we would be successful. I believed that to the core of my being.

I had to focus and start narrowing down researched options.
We were still waiting to have our oncology appointment here in
Canada, but my gut instinct told me we would have to travel out of
the country. Friends and acquaintances alike would reach out with
recommendations. I had no idea how to sift through them all or
understand which might benefit Terri the most.

Then I reminded myself to trust my instincts. Even present day, I
am still learning to trust my instincts on the big and small things.
The other day while at the hospital for work I walked into the
bathroom and was debating which stall to enter. I thought to
myself that I shouldn't go in the middle stall, but brushed the
thought away thinking that it was silly. I went into the stall, and
I looked over a little too late to realize that there was no toilet
paper. It was another nudge to remind me how well we can be
guided along our path in an easier manner if we just trust our
innate wisdom. Trust, trust, trust.

There were three options that I was ultimately being drawn to,
one was a clinic in Mexico focusing on the Gerson Therapy, one
a clinic in Germany focusing on Nanoknife, and a third clinic in
Austria focusing on Immunotherapy and Hyperthermia.

At that time, my knowledge of what could be done procedurally
was very limited and I had no idea whether Terri would be eligible
for surgery. A friend sent me a news article about the mayor
of Toronto raising funds to travel to Germany to this clinic for
Nanoknife treatment. Essentially, as stated on the Nanoknife
website, it is an: "Ablation procedure that involved the delivery of
a series of high voltage direct current electrical pulses between
two electrodes placed within a target area of tissue."

I was enthusiastic about this procedure, so I completed all the
paperwork and the application form and sent it off to Germany. At
the same time, I ordered books on the Gerson Therapy, innovative
cancer treatments; by that time the kids were on their way home
from school, and some much-needed family time was a priority.

To be honest, during this time we spoke to a friend whose sister
had travelled to the clinic in Austria. We asked some questions

and it seemed like an option, but it was not something we pursued further in that moment. In our overwhelmed state, the information did not quite register; although, the seed was planted.

A Lesson in Strategy

As I lay in bed that night, I kept thinking about what Terri's cancer might need. How are we possibly going to conquer all of these tumors? I had such destructive words in my thoughts—we wanted to kill the cancer. Destroy it. Eviscerate it. I wanted it gone. Every single ounce of it.

Visualizing through all of my senses and the colours of the rainbow, I entered my workshop in MindScape. I was so happy and appreciative to be there. I instantly felt the most calming wave of sensations, and before I invited Terri in for a healing, I enjoyed a walk through my nature area into a forest. My dog Jukie accompanied me, and I strategized over what I thought might be the best strategies to help Terri.

Those dangerous and destructive words were penetrating through the layers of my mind, and I felt in that moment that we needed to destroy the cancer. It popped in my head clear as day—why not simply remove the cancer? I knew that it would not be on an energetic level alone—but trusted that starting to work on that layer would allow the effects to be felt in physical reality.

I invited Terri into my Mindscape, and he marveled at my workshop. He wanted to spend time exploring once again, and this time he was mesmerized by the fountain of life which was a beautiful waterfall guests would see immediately after entering through my elevator. It was the purest of water, a healing source of energy, and before I could say anything Terri leaped right in. It was incredible to watch—rainbows formed around him, dancing from within him, and light radiated from his body refracting off every corner of my workshop. To me, that represented his willingness to be in my workshop, and demonstrated that his chakras were working to align from the healing water.

In my healing room, I told him that I meant business. I explained how I thought it would be best if we tossed his cancer right into the garbage. I had to get to it first though, so I drilled holes in his stomach, pulled his organs out of his body, and laid them on the table. In such a calculated manner, I pulled every little piece of cancer out of his pancreas, liver, lymph nodes and stomach that I could see. I threw it in my trash can, and then incinerated it.

I felt very productive, and once I placed all of Terri's organs back inside of him, we cuddled up and went to sleep. Not being used to accessing my alpha mind yet, I found that Mindscape was both invigorating and exhausting, so I fell asleep quickly and had another fabulous sleep. What a gift that was!

In the morning when we woke, Terri stretched and then cringed in pain. Not used to feeling symptoms of the cancer, and quickly recalling that the work I had done on him the previous day had impacted him physically, he asked, "Did you work on me again last night?"

Seeing the half appreciative grin, but pain in his eyes as he held his side, I slowly responded, "Yeeeesssss. I honestly thought I was helping. I am so sorry if somehow I have caused you some discomfort."

"Perhaps you could stop using such invasive tactics?" He half joked.

We went on with our day, but I really spent time letting those words sink in. I understood the benefits of MindScape, how we could overcome physical barriers and heal and grow in unlimited ways—so what was I doing wrong?

I reached out to my instructor Kristin and let her know what had happened. How I had offered two healings to Terri in my MindScape, and he had felt both on the physical level, but not necessarily in the most positive way.

She offered the most profound piece of advice that changed the way we viewed MindScape, cancer, and essentially life.

"When in life does it ever serve us to fight something?" she questioned. "Instead of fighting the cancer, why do you not try to love it? Understand it? Learn from it—why is it there, and what is it trying to show you?"

I thanked Kristin for her advice and fell to the floor in tears. I felt almost as overwhelmed as the moment when we found out about Terri's diagnosis. Had I been approaching this all wrong? It made so much sense though—when does fighting something ever work? Does it ever bring you farther ahead in your health, or a relationship? That is what you hear though- this person is fighting cancer, that person is fighting Parkinson's…. the references are endless.

The light switch turned on. If every physical symptom is coming from an awareness that our mind is bringing to our attention, why not embrace it? In order to overcome the symptom/disease/barrier, we must learn from it and understand why it is truly there. We wanted to move forward, and in order to do so we needed to do the work. We wanted to grow. Most of all, we wanted Terri to heal.

From that moment forward we stopped fighting the cancer. We chose to love it, understand it, and grow from it. Never again did I cause any physical discomfort to Terri because I completely modified my healings. Truth be told, I would not say that Terri fully embraced loving his cancer, which is completely understandable. However, he was open to learning and growing from it.

What would happen if we all shifted our perceptions? Opened our minds to the profound possibility of new beginnings. We could say goodbye to the disease, loneliness, weight, addictions—whatever it may be. Just imagine for a moment the shift we would see if we took time to understand their presence. What brought these symptoms from our mind to our physical presence? What do we need to do to learn, grow and overcome them?

It is all possible. Healing, change, dreams coming to reality, and unlimited possibilities. Never give up. Rather than fight, choose to embrace.

Chapter

LETTING GO OF THE RAGE

The road was winding, and I sighed deeply as I traced hearts into the passenger window of Terri's truck. The terrain made it difficult to speed as you could not even see around the next bend. It was a different sort of mountain to admire, the deep valleys surrounding Drumheller molded with character, sharp edges and a miraculous sort of peace.

At that moment, I wished that some of that serene peace could be transferred to me. Trying hard not to let the argument escalate in front of the kids, it was quickly becoming the most difficult battle I had ever tried to win.

Vienna, Austria is where we should head for treatment. I knew it in my heart, my soul and from the tips of my fingers to the tips of my toes; I just did. As I explored all the clinics, I was constantly drawn back to Dr. Kleef and his clinic in Austria. His successes, treatment plan, demeanor and knowledge were all incredibly alluring. I reminisced back to the moment when Terri was diagnosed. Once the tears passed, I said "You are now my husband and my project, and I will not take less than an A++."

The tears were welling as Terri yelled that he did not want to go to Austria. I had to stop arguing; I knew it was only going to get worse, nor would it solve anything. My heart ached—how do I convince my husband that he needs to go there? I completely understood that it was not his rational mind saying no, but rather his ego trying to protect him. According to his ego, going to Austria was not a safe decision. It was radical, consequential, and full of impact. A decision that could result in saving his life. I needed plan B, and I knew what it would entail. Luckily, we were en route to the destination where I could make it happen.

Saskatchewan was our home for most of our lives, and we were heading back to see our families, and attend a fundraiser for Terri that was spearheaded by fabulous friends and our community. We had not officially made the decision yet where we were going for treatment, but we knew it was going to be expensive stepping outside of traditional Western Medical care.

As the drive went on, we all took turns closing our eyes, snacking and playing silly car games. We laughed and laughed as the memory game started with, "What would you bring with you on a trip to Mexico?" Rather than a bathing suit or toothbrush, the kids would suggest a trampoline, watermelon, or the backseat of the car. That would be interesting to try and explain to customs!

We arrived at Terri's parents' house and changed for the fundraiser. We had no idea what to expect, who would be there, or more importantly the magnitude of the experience. It brings tears to my eyes when I recall walking through those front doors.

Arriving at Hudson's Bar, we opened the front door and were greeted by good friends and family. Once I turned the corner, I could not believe my eyes. I held Terri's hand tightly and braced myself. The entire bar was full of guests attending the fundraiser. There were hundreds of people there.

Not only that, but the silent auction items they gathered for the event were awe-inspiring. You often see bottles of wine, or a certificate for a massage. They had pulled together items that were off the charts. There was a hot tub for silent auction, a golf trip to the US, incredible prize baskets, and an Edmonton Oilers jersey signed by Mark Messier.

Terri and I separated for most of the night, spending time touring around the bar trying to socialize with everyone. Not only were all of the guests reeling from Terri's diagnosis as we were, but we had moved to Calgary a year earlier and had a lot of catching up to do with many familiar faces.

At times during the evening, I felt overwhelmed with tears. Others, I felt like I was floating around the room taking deep breaths trying to ground myself. It was akin to being at our wedding again, trying to be so respectful and ensure that everyone was acknowledged. Trying to feel gratitude for seeing all of the wonderful faces was overshadowed by the fact that we were not there, in that moment, to celebrate joy. We were there to fundraise to save a life: Terri's life. My beautiful husband's life.

Throughout the evening, I had a very deliberate message to share with guests. Each of my one-on-one conversations, especially with Terri's core group of friends, was light chit chat followed by a clear directive. "Please tell Terri he needs to go to Austria. It may be too hard to digest coming from me, but he needs to hear it tonight.

From you, from all, with magnitude."

Later, I overheard Terri talking with his best friend, and I could slightly make out snippets of the conversation.

"What do you have to lose?" Deke asked. He stood face to face with Terri, two hands on his shoulders. I saw Terri's head bow and tears well in his eyes. It was what needed to be said. It was what he needed to hear. Deke's words clearly resonated with the message that I had been trying to drive home to Terri—that there was nothing to lose and everything to gain.

The moment came at the fundraiser where we had to acknowledge our guests publicly. I do not remember what exactly Terri and I said, I only recall a brief part of my speech that went something like this:

"It is amazing that you have all gathered here to support this most magnificent man. He has brought joy, laughter and memories to each one of us in this room. I can say one thing with certainty— the next time that we gather all together, it will be to celebrate that Terri Mah is cancer free."

The crowd applauded, and we cried. I absolutely felt it in my heart. I trusted it then and trust it now; as I remind Terri, I signed up for *at least* 50 years of marriage, not ten. The kids have heard that phrase a few times, and they needed to make sure that the *at least* was included.

As the evening concluded, we left emotionally drained, inspired, and completely overwhelmed. We could never have dreamt of our community showing up like that for us. The gratitude we hold in our hearts for that evening is eternal. We feel so much appreciation for all those who contributed, and they will never be forgotten. Hudson's said it had been their largest fundraiser in history. We were so incredibly blessed.

A New Day

As we went to bed that night, I let the Austria discussion rest. We just cuddled and prayed for strength and the ability to make the right decisions.

The kids were up bright and early the following morning to enjoy grandma's eggs and bacon. I took the luxury of having a nice long shower, while Terri listened to one of his BodyTalk sessions from my friend. I learned later that in that session Terri had released the most profound emotion of rage. Not anger, it was so much deeper than that. It was pure, unfiltered rage. Rage about why this was happening to him, rage about the impact it had on his family, and rage about whether healing was possible.

When an emotion like that is so stuck, it can impede any facet of our bodymind complex—physical, emotional or mental. Although I did not put the pieces together until later, that session may have been one of the most crucial he would ever have.

You see, while I was sitting out on the terrace at grandma's, I decided it was time. There would be no more messing around— we needed to determine a treatment plan and act on it.

I sipped my coffee and took a moment to enjoy the simplicities of life. A sip of coffee can seem like magic with its calming effect. Terri came out onto the terrace, and I looked up from my coffee. The kids were off playing, so I knew that this was an opportune moment. If we were going to argue about this, it was perfect that we were alone.

"We are going to Austria," I stated. "I believe that the clinic there has the most incredible treatment plan I have found anywhere in the world."

"God guided me to find this clinic, Terri." I calmly asserted. "Not only that, our daughter's name is Vienna," I cracked a tiny smile. You know, the kind where only the corners of your mouth curl up. "If that is not a sign from the Divine, I do not know what is."

I was ready for a battle in response, but took a deep breath and said, "I'm booking it today. Flights, apartment, all of it. We are going as a family."

The silence seemed like an eternity as I paused for a response from Terri. He simply shrugged his shoulders and agreed, "Okay." That was it. One simple word that would change our future, aid in curing his cancer and give us back our destiny.

I could not believe it. Later I understood just how much of an impact letting go of that rage had on Terri. It freed his mind to be open to new possibilities.

Imagine if we all took the time to dig through those deep emotional layers what new possibilities could awaken in all of us? We can manifest our entire destiny; it is those difficult steps, our ego protecting us that we need to challenge. Thank you, ego for protecting me and bringing me to this moment of time. Let's see what else we can discover together; I am ready for some expansion. Funny how when we take a moment to acknowledge the thought, or the way our egos are limiting us, then move past that barrier. The same type of realization we had when we awakened to the knowledge that we were not going to win by trying to fight the cancer. We needed to become coherent with it, understand it, and try to decipher the messages it was bringing.

This book is not solely about the true story of Terri beating Stage IV Pancreatic Cancer. It's about courage, hope and returning to those childhood dreams wherein we thought the world was our oyster, and the imagination we painted in our minds of our future was full of vivid colours, depth and pure joy. The reality is that those dreams were never intended to become stagnant in our childhood. Get back there—dream big, heal big, live big. The world is our oyster. Today, tomorrow and every day.

The sun set and the planning began. It was another day and another step towards a new direction. Giving us a future. Giving Terri hope. My canvas was once again starting to represent an outcome of joy, love and the complete gratitude we had for each other and our family. I will cherish that moment, that simple word *okay,* as one of the most instrumental in my entire life.

Chapter

THERE HE WAS JUST A WALKIN' DOWN THE STREET

Handing over our boarding passes and passports felt oddly reminiscent of a family vacation. We often travelled to Mexico and enjoyed endless hours playing catch in the pool, and devouring nachos, fresh guacamole and virgin Bahama Mamas. The airport had the same smell, the same look, but the ambience around us felt oh-so-different. I kept checking over my shoulder as we walked the catwalk to the airplane, as I felt the energy emerging—there was so much love and support there. I will never have proof, but my soul said we were being followed, and carried by a whole host of angels—carrying us towards new beginnings, and not towards endings. I could sense those angles lifting us to challenge our thoughts, our capabilities and enhance our momentum. Giving us arms of safety. I looked over my shoulder one last time before we stepped onto the plane, and I swear I saw my dad's face in the energy of angels. I sighed, smiled, and focused my attention back on my children as we boarded.

Childhood wonder transformed Nixon and Vienna's faces as we took our seats. "There are so many rows!"; "We both get to be by the window!"; "I love the colors!"; "Mom, mom, mom—look! There are blankets on our seat for us!"

It was the most wonderful way for us to begin our trip. To the kids it was not a trip to save daddy's life, it was an adventure. No different than going to Mexico. As we buckled, I reached behind to hold Terri's hand. "That is how I am going to treat it as well," I thought. A God given adventure to make us stronger—as individuals and as a family. It would have been so easy for us to board that plane allowing fear and panic to overcome us. It was a choice to choose fear or choose gratitude. We are far from perfect at it, but to this day we do our best to choose gratitude, embrace the moment and love the opportunity. As Eckhart Tolle says:

Some changes look negative on the surface, but you will soon realize that space is being created in your life for something new to emerge.

How would your life transform if you chose to see any hardship you are facing as an opportunity to grow? In that moment I felt like Terri was a caterpillar, and his treatment, deep diving into consciousness and finding new perspective was going to help him emerge as the most incredibly beautiful and magnificent butterfly ever seen. It was going to be our journey together. I was ready for us to transform alongside him and become a family of butterflies.

Sweet Dreams

Air Austria was flying us direct from Calgary to Frankfurt, the kids' first ever overnight flight. Their service and meals were incredible, and they catered to our gluten free requests without question.

Once we had eaten, enjoyed some screen time and the late hours were bringing on yawns, we snuggled our little munchkins up as best as we could. We were hoping to get a few hours of rest before we landed in Europe.

As I closed my eyes, I slowed my breathing and allowed myself to go into MindScape. I enjoyed every moment there, knowing that once I allowed myself back into the Alpha state of mind, that is where true change and growth can happen.

This time though I was only wanting to observe. When I entered my workshop, I instantly felt so at ease. Entirely at peace. I laid down in my healing room, and without prompting, a movie started playing in front of me. The title appeared, *A Moment in Time.* I giggled, not knowing what the moment was that was going to unveil itself before me, but I trusted it would be perfect.

My Second Home

It was springtime in Sevilla, Spain and the streets were bustling with people. Kids had just arrived home from school, and a lot of young adults were enjoying their siesta hours before returning to work for the evening shift.

I had been in Spain for eight months by this point and had overcome the language barriers. It was my goal to become fluent in Spanish—read it, write it and speak it. By far, it was the steepest learning curve I had been through in my twenty-five years, but overcoming great challenges always felt so rewarding.

The day I had packed my bag to go to Spain, I stood on Terri's front step and we awkwardly shared one last hug. We knew that the connection between us was deep and lasting, and we murmured a shy *I love you* under our breaths. There was no way I wasn't going to Spain though, becoming fluent was one of the biggest items on my bucket list.

Here we were eight months later, and Terri was coming to visit me. The family I was nannying for kindly allowed Terri to stay with us, they even gave me a week off to vacation with him.
I had no idea what to expect. I'm not sure I had ever been nervous, wondering how it was going to feel to see his face after all this time, to hold his hand, and enjoy his company.

The movie flashed back to a million phone calls, as Terri and I had grown closer than ever over those eight months. He was getting on with life as normal in Canada, casually dating and enjoying his career. But we would talk every day—I mean every single day, and for at least an hour. With the time change we would squeeze in a quick call before he headed to work in the morning, and I would often call him in the middle of the night when I returned home from one of my dancing escapades. I had made so many wonderful friends but was never more excited than to pick up the phone and tell Terri about my day. He would even listen to me trying to read Spanish, struggling to pronounce the words, or attempting to conjugate verbs.

Sebastian and Ines, the wonderful kids I was nannying, were with me so Terri had to take a cab out from Sevilla to Montequinto, the town where my host family lived. The tears welled up in my eyes as the movie played out before me. It was the most intense anticipation I had ever felt in my life.

The kids and I were standing on one side of the street, and I saw a cab stopping across from us on the other side. We took a step back as a bus roared up in front of us, and a swarm of passengers filed off. The anticipation in my heart surged, and I dodged left to right adjusting my view around the bus to see if that was him. Had my Terri arrived?

The bus pulled away, and in the same instance I saw the cab driver pull away. Was that him? I squinted to reframe my perception, and I quickly saw a hand waving and smiling. My heart raced and I pointed to the corner where the nearest cross walk was outlined. It was Terri! He was here—to see me. He was here for us, for this opportunity for us!

I waited on the corner and I could not still my feet. They danced with enthusiasm as I beamed with a smile. There he was! Wait a minute though—there was something quite different about him. He looked radiant, fresh, and completely healthy looking.

Clearly, he was not honest about what else he had been up to at home. He had been working out like crazy. I was already in love with this man, and on top of it all, he now looked like a supermodel. My heart swelled so big; I quickly tried to fix my hair wondering if his perception of me was anything alike my own.

When he made it to my side of the street, I collapsed into his arms. My heart was full. I did not know in that moment the incredible destiny that God had in store for us, but I did know that I had never been more in love in my life.

As the movie continued to play out, I enjoyed watching our journey through Spain together; getting lost while looking for the city of Marbella (this was long before Google Maps), and driving up this tiny road around a cliffside mountain, only to nearly run over someone's pet donkey tied to a tree. It was quite a memorable sight!

I laughed out loud and then caught myself trying not to wake the kids. Clear as day, the movie played. Terri and I were on a plane flying to Ibiza for our romantic weekend. If you are not familiar with it, Ibiza is an incredibly trendy and happening city in Spain. As we sat on the plane, I rolled my eyes at Terri's outfit. He was wearing double pleated, skinny black corduroy pants that were two sizes too big. His choice of shirt was plain white and by no means fashionable. The neck was stretched out and looked like it had been awkwardly hung on a hanger a few times. There was a pocket on the left front side of the shirt, with a tiny mustard stain running along the seam.

When we were getting ready for dinner at the hotel that night, I sat on Terri's lap and tried to keep it lighthearted. "Okay," I said.

"You look absolutely incredible: so handsome! I just cannot let you do it. I have to be honest—you are too good looking to dress like this anymore."

He laughed and shrugged his shoulders, clearly not taking offence to my comment but knowing there was some truth to it. "Shopping isn't my strong suit," he said with a smirk. With a little tickle and a kiss on the neck, he smiled, "What are you going to do about it?" he teased.

"I will show you!" I laughed and started running around the room. "Hmm," I stated. "I guess you will need a couple of things for the short term. The rest has got to go!"

With that, I laid a pair of jeans and a couple of slightly plausible shirts on the bed. I took the rest and confidently walked over to the garbage. I smushed his clothes into the garbage can and looked at him with anticipation.

I was half expecting anger, or at least a frown. It took me by surprise to see an enormous smile slowly spread across his face. We started laughing hysterically, and he shrugged, "Alright, I guess you are taking me shopping then."

———◆———

A New Country

I woke to the sound of Vienna poking me on the plane. "Mom, are you awake?"

"I am now," I thought. "Mom, I love you… when are we going to land?"

I was happy to see that we had all slept a solid number of hours, and that the flight attendants were coming around with breakfast delivery service.

As we enjoyed our breakfast, played word games and coloured, I felt so much gratitude for the movie that played in my Mindscape before I had drifted off. Never would I have imagined that our life would take us here, but somehow, I just knew it would be okay.

We were ready to do the work, take the plunge, and step into that new chapter. Just as Terri was ready to shed his outdated clothing when he visited me in Spain, he was now ready to shed the layers of active memories, fear and pain that had created this cancer. I was ready to be right there with him. Not just to watch or encourage him, but to do the work alongside him and heal some of my inner shadows.

Now looking back at the plane ride, we had no idea what our experience in Austria would be like, or how we would feel. My instincts brought us there. Scientists now say that our instincts are our strongest form of intelligence. For me, it is our connection to the God-given energy around us and through us, that shows us signs and propels us to where we need to be. Our instincts are showing us our path. Trust them, use them and listen to them. The more you do, the stronger they become. Imagine if we all stopped letting our egos prevent us from growth and change, and let our instincts guide the way to the profound healing, life changing, incredible experiences that wait for us to be brave enough to find them once we are ready to step outside of the box. Oh, wait a minute—whoever said there was a box in the first place? Trust yourself, do the work—take down those boundaries that are holding you back from your true destiny. There may be some hard times along the way as it does take courage to do the work, but the rewards are boundless, on all levels—physical, mental, emotional, spiritual. A whole new destiny awaits you. You must be willing to dive in.

Chapter

WELCOME TO AUSTRIA

The sun set and the breeze from the street carried the humidity of a hot Vienna day. Our apartment was near the Schonbrun palace and zoo which we were excited to explore during our stay. Renting an apartment seemed to be the most affordable option for our time spent in Vienna, however the only thing that seemed to be missing was air conditioning. It was evening and still a scorching thirty-five degrees Celsius outside.

There was a beautiful, quaint grocery store around the corner where we stocked up on groceries. For a small store, they had a good selection of gluten-free products, and the kids were so excited to see the giant fresh orange juicer. Like kids in a candy store, they would drop orange after orange into the juicer and fill a bottle large enough for both to share.

We made the mistake of having an afternoon nap once we landed, as they recommend staying awake until evening time. Since we were awake anyway, we took the opportunity to explore once we unloaded our groceries.

According to Google maps we were less than a ten-minute walk from Dr. Kleef's clinic, and we wanted to make sure we knew exactly how to get there, so our trek would be nice and simple in the morning.

The subway station was just across the corner from our apartment, and we took a moment to show the kids the subway map and how it all worked. They were intrigued, and very excited to ride the train in the upcoming weeks. From there we strolled down a residential street, holding hands and skipping along. There were a few little boutique shops, and you could see the kids processing the difference between a Canadian residential street and a European one. They commented on the cobblestone street, and how bumpy it would be to drive on. They laughed at how the mopeds and scooters were parked on top of each other and crammed together. Nixon loved the greenery of the beautiful trees, and Vienna wondered when she would be able to purchase a shirt with *Vienna* printed on it.

On our way, we found a gorgeous park-like setting and it had a subtle but quaint white gazebo in the corner. It resembled the perfect setting for our first family picture in Austria. We approached the gates and soon realized it was a restaurant. The kids jumped up and down proclaiming how starving they were, and we giggled knowing there was no way that was true. It was early in the evening and mealtime somewhere, we thought, still processing the time change.

Unfortunately, the famous Austrian wiener schnitzel was not gluten free at this restaurant, but that did not seem to bother anyone. We dined on spiced potatoes, delicious sausage and salad. We chatted about all the things we were going to explore in Austria after a good night's sleep. Terri and I squeezed hands under the table, with an unspoken hopefulness that we would be able to maintain the idea to the kids that this was as much of a family vacation and experience as it was treatment for Terri.

We ended our dinner with a family photo under the beautiful gazebo and carried on finding Dr. Kleef's clinic.

As we approached the address, we came across the most interesting intersection. There were four winding roads weaving in every which direction, and a roundabout in the middle. As we tried to understand where we should cross the street, we realized that at the high point of the intersection was Dr. Kleef's office. The white office building stood tall and proud, at the head of this conglomerate of roads, and it felt so inviting it took my breath away. My instincts overtook me at that moment, and I whispered to Terri, "You are going to be okay." He smiled and gave me a kiss on the forehead.

Even now, remembering that moment brings me such a sense of gratitude and warmth in my heart. An eternal appreciation for God's guidance and direction that led us down the right path.

<hr>

Welcome to the Clinic

We were not quite ready to wake in the morning to return to meet Dr. Kleef at his office, but we stretched, yawned, and all slowly rolled out of bed. We talked about how cool it was that we were waking up in a different country, and continent (that took some explaining), and how back at our home in Canada it would still be the middle of the night.

"Would Jukie still be sleeping?" Vienna asked. Our sweet puppy, Jukie, was staying with our family who were so kind to look after her.

"Yes, sweetie. I'm sure that she is having sweet puppy dreams about bully sticks and her ball." We laughed and talked about how whenever you give Jukie a treat, she hauls it to the living room floor and announces who is boss. She dances, barks and plays with the treat before finally deciding to eat it. This is our family's favorite Jukie-watching moment.

When we arrived at Dr. Kleef's building, I had that same momentous feeling. I realized that my left hand was quivering a little, and my heart was starting to race. We opened the door to the building and looked at the directory. Third Floor. Wonderful, I thought. Another sign—on the floor of my all-time favorite number.

The spiral staircase to the third floor was beautifully classic. Not well adorned, just simple enough to allow you to appreciate its structural design. At the top of the stairs, we opened the doorway into Dr. Kleef's office. I almost wanted to collapse. I felt such an anticipation and admiration for a man I had not even personally met yet. I had read enough to understand his vision and simply admired how bold he was to step out of the norm, challenge the traditional Western Medical system, and provide hope to those who may otherwise feel lost.

There was no one at the front desk, so we stood patiently and waited. My eyes scanned the rooms, and I noticed that the clinic was quaint. It did not feel like a hospital, or sterile in any manner. I smelled a subtle scent of orange, and I admired the herringbone patterned hardwood flooring. I smiled, thinking that this was just another sign. It was my dream to have herringbone flooring, in my mind it was the classiest and most profoundly bold flooring pattern you could choose. "Profoundly bold," I thought. That is what we are—profoundly bold in this journey. Profoundly bold in being brave enough to challenge Terri's body and both of our minds to grow, change, and release those limiting belief systems that have manifested into pain and dis-ease.

I snapped out of my daydream when a lovely young lady greeted us from the desk. Her accent was stunning, as she welcomed us to the clinic. After introductions were completed, she guided us to the waiting room.

As we passed the time, the kids took great interest in the coffee machine, offering to make us tea. There were colouring books, and a fish tank full of cute fish. I have no idea how long we were in the waiting room: it felt as though time stood still.

Before I knew it, the lovely nurse had returned, and she asked us to accompany her to Dr. Kleef's office. His office was a beautiful corner office with windows overlooking two sides of the neighborhood below. There was a table in the back, and two chairs facing Dr. Kleef's desk. Before we sat, we all shook Dr. Kleef's hand and introduced ourselves.

———————————◆————————————

Cuddles and Plans

Later, back at the apartment, we kissed the kids and talked about all of the fun things we were going to explore in Austria. They had amazing outdoor pools, koala bears and panda bears at the zoo, and churches galore. We had read about the beautiful churches, including the magnificent St. Stephen's Cathedral downtown. We were ever so conscious not to focus on the CT scan Terri was going to have the next day, along with blood work and other testing. Dr. Kleef was insisted on all of Terri's vital information to be up to date for his detailed plan of attack. Or as we would call it, a detailed plan of understanding the cancer, and asking it kindly to step aside.

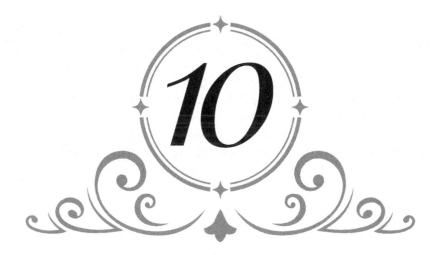

Chapter

10

DR. RALF KLEEF

With the powerful belief that your body has an amazing ability to heal, Dr. Kleef has created his treatments and therapies following in the footsteps of William B. Coley, renowned as the father of cancer immunotherapy.

Dr. Kleef's clinic focuses on individualized diagnostics and cancer immunotherapy. His treatment plan is entirely specialized and dependent on a particular patient and his illness. Based on years of experience and a profound passion for immunotherapy, his approach is unparalleled.

The clinic was founded in 1998 and has demonstrated revolutionary success over two decades. As years passed, Dr. Kleef focused on new techniques and continually expanded his awareness in this field. Many patients have experienced incredible success at his clinic, and we are blessed to be among them. We are bold in our advocacy of Dr. Kleef's treatment regimens and their adaptability. We strongly recommend that any individual facing cancer of any type, or battling chronic disease, should reach out to Dr. Kleef to determine whether his treatment plan would be a good fit.

————————◆————————

Dr. Kleef's History

The information on the following pages is from Dr. Kleef's website:

Dr. Ralf Kleef has an extensive list of qualifications, dating back when he accomplished his state examinations in medicine at the University of Witten-Herdecke, Germany in 1991. Beyond that, he also became an ND, specializing in naturopathic medicine. It all came together with his training in Hyperthermia, and in 2004 he was appointed by the courts as Sworn court certified expert for hyperthermia and Complimentary Medicine.

In addition, Dr. Kleef also specialized in immunology at the Memorial Sloan Kettering Cancer Center in New York City, and discovered the benefit of combining all these treatments with immunotherapy. As a young doctor, Dr. Kleef was also very fortunate to be part of a clinic in Germany that was one of the first that utilized hyperthermia to treat cancer. Incorporating this foundation with Dr. Coley's methodologies, Dr. Kleef was ready to put his research into practice. Coupled with an extraordinary passion to save lives and change the face of modern medicine, Dr. Kleef was bound to be a success and a blessing to the world of medicine.

Foundations of Treatment- Hyperthermia and Immunotherapy

At Dr. Kleef Hyperthermie, the foundation of treatment is based on an analysis of the human organism itself. Dr. Kleef says the body alone is the mentor for treatments. The core regimen of the treatment plan is hyperthermia, and by accelerating the body's temperature it allows the body to help itself and accelerate sustainable recovery.

Hyperthermia

Hyperthermia, by definition, is the targeted increase of the body's core temperature. Considered to be one of the most effective therapies in physical medicine, it is the core foundation of Dr. Kleef's treatment. Due to its effectiveness and the profound results of hyperthermia, the Deutsche Krebshilfe (also known as the German Cancer Aid Organization), it has now been dubbed the *fourth weapon against cancer.*

In a hyperthermia treatment, a medical device is utilized in order to heat the tumorous tissues from the outside to a temperature of 43 degrees Celsius. This is accomplished through high-frequency radio waves which deplete the tumor of both oxygen and nutrients, creating an acidic environment within which the tumor cell cannot function. The fascinating part is that the skin and outer layers of tissue are not damaged by the heat. In addition, hyperthermia also has a positive impact on the immune system as the heat causes the cancer cells to look different to the body than normal tissue. The heat assists in bringing awareness to the immune system and the body that the cancerous cells need to be destroyed. The devices utilized to accomplish this are one of the following:

1- Deep-Hyperthermia Oncotherm EHY2000
2- Deep-Hyperthermia Synchotherm RF600T

Immunotherapy

Hyperthermia is combined with immunotherapy for maximum results. In Dr. Kleef's words, immunotherapy is *experiencing a global renaissance*. Immunotherapy activates your T-cells, more specifically referred to as so-called Checkpoint inhibitors (PDL-1/PD-1 and CTL4 antibodies) and has provided options for cancers that were previously deemed incurable.

Immunotherapy works to strengthen the body's immune system so that it can target the areas of cancer more effectively. Like a light switch for T-cells, it helps keep them *turned on* to do their job.

Whole-Body Hyperthermia

The final piece to the trifecta of treatment is the combination of these checkpoint inhibitors with local, regional and whole-body hyperthermia combined with an immunotherapy, named interleukin 2 (IL-2). More commonly referred to by patients as *fever week,* it is important to be reminded that fever is not a disease; alternatively, it works to strengthen the immune system and is a natural defense against bacteria and viruses.

There is an abundance of documentation on the success of fever treatment, and in 1900, it began to demonstrate success in cancer therapy as well. Dr. William Coley was the pioneer of using fever-causing agents with cancer and with that he demonstrated remarkable success. Dr. Kleef gained some of these foundational ideas from Dr. Coley and transformed them into modern day practice.

Dr. Kleef analyzes each patient in his clinic consistently, and on a frequent basis, to make sure schedules, agendas and dosages are enough to set the individual up for success. Other regimens are often included and will be discussed in further detail in the chapter outlining Terri's personalized treatment at the clinic.

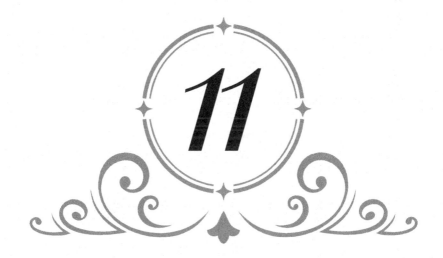

Chapter

CT #2 WAS A SHOCKER

We were starting to get accustomed to Vienna, and the kids and I were enjoying our time there. After only a few days, Nixon had mastered the subway lines and could easily direct us home from one area of the city or another. Riding the subway was such a novel thrill; one day we went all the way across town just to enjoy what was the city's best ice cream. To some this may have seemed a frivolous waste of time, but for us we were simply enjoying every family moment together. An ice cream treat that may have taken only a few minutes to devour turned into an afternoon adventure of sunshine, subways and togetherness. Imagine if we all changed our perceptions to enjoy the simple things in life—the small moments, the journey and the destination with an *embrace every moment* kind of attitude. With such an attitude of love and gratitude, would that not in itself transform our physical, mental and emotional health?

Oncology Appointment #2

As we strolled into Dr. Kleef's office for our first official consultation where a treatment plan would be developed, Terri and I could not hide the distress on our faces.

"What's wrong mommy?" Vienna asked politely.

"Nothing sweetheart," I replied. "Mom and dad are just anxious to hear what Dr. Kleef has to tell us today."

"Okay, mommy—may I sit over here and colour?"

"Absolutely you can my love." Vienna set up with some crayons and asked me a few more questions about what I would like her to draw.

Without hesitation Nixon pulled a chair from the table up to the desk. It was clear that the *big boy at the table* feeling was not something he was willing to let go of anytime soon. It was adorable.

Dr. Kleef walked elegantly into his office wearing such a warm and welcoming smile. Standing tall and proud, his confidence instantly gave me hope. He acknowledged the kids with a smile and said, "Hello Mahs. How are we today?" We all answered politely and patiently waited as he logged onto his computer.

Instinctively, I trusted him. I only knew his reputation and had skimmed the surface of his methodologies and approaches, but in that moment my confidence in our decision to come to Vienna felt certain. It felt right. It was not my brain providing me this information, but those Spidey senses we all have; the most profound gift we are all born with to guide us through our life: our instincts. My instincts reminded me that we were exactly where we needed to be. I did not know why as we still did not have any answers from Terri's blood work or his CT scan, but I took a deep breath and knew to trust. "Thank you, God, for bringing us to this time and place. We are grateful." I silently prayed these words to God as Dr. Kleef opened his computer and started looking through Terri's results.

In the same instant, by acknowledging the moment with gratitude, I was hoping to diminish the thoughts that were trying to creep in. "What if the CT is worse? What if he tells us that treatment will not work? How will we feel if we came all this way for nothing?" I took a deep breath and thanked the thoughts for being there but that I chose to re-focus on different thoughts: positive, loving, life changing, healing thoughts. As soon as I reminded myself of this, my heart rate slowed, and I focused back on my external world. I noticed that Dr. Kleef had read Terri's file, and then took a moment to refocus and read again. He put his glasses on and looked perplexed.

We sat patiently as we waited for Dr. Kleef's words, "What sort of treatment did you do in Canada before you came here?" he asked.

Terri replied that he had completed one dose of chemo, 2 IV-Vitamin C treatments, and approximately 30 BodyTalk sessions. Terri also went on to explain that the one dose of chemo (before I had convinced him to stop), was done shortly before we travelled to Austria, so he did not think that it would have taken effect yet. Of course, there was no explanation required for what IV Vitamin C was, as that was an integral part of Dr. Kleef's treatment at the clinic.

"What is BodyTalk?" Dr. Kleef patiently asked.

Terri looked at me to answer, and I was wondering why in this moment would I need to be explaining BodyTalk? There was something on that computer screen that was bringing up these questions for Dr. Kleef. I knew that BodyTalk was most of the treatment that Terri had received thus far, and I also confidently knew that BodyTalk could never do any harm. I started to feel a tingle run through my body: a tingle of hope, a feeling of life, and an overwhelming sense of optimism.

When explaining to individuals and medical professionals who are not familiar with BodyTalk, I always try to keep it as simple as possible.

"BodyTalk is energy healing, Dr. Kleef. Rather than just looking at only physical symptoms, it looks at the whole picture of how the physical, emotional, mental, and spiritual, are all connected." I paused to see if this was enough of an explanation in the moment. "Oh yes," replied Dr. Kleef. "I have heard of things like this, maybe called something else."

"Absolutely," I replied. "There are many forms of energy healing." I stopped myself from going any further as I really wanted to know what Dr. Kleef had seen in Terri's report!

Dr. Kleef looked away from the computer screen and directly at us. He took his glasses off and a kind smile spread across his face.

"Well," he said. "This is rather unusual and quite impressive. You are already in partial remission."

Terri and I looked at each other as we tried to process the words, he was saying.

"Partial remission?" Terri asked with a squeak in his voice.

"Yes!" replied Dr. Kleef.

"What does that mean?" Nixon asked. Dr. Kleef smiled again, acutely aware of the fact that our children were in the room with us, and he was very talented at modifying his language so as not to intimidate them.

Dr. Kleef turned the computer screen towards us and explained what he was seeing.

"In your original CT," he explained, "you had one tumor in your pancreas, two tumors in your lymph nodes, one in your stomach, and over 20 lesions in your liver."

"What this shows is that the tumor in the pancreas is gone, and the two tumors in the lymph nodes are gone. I am not sure how you did it, but before you begin treatment here you are already in partial remission."

The rest of the conversation seemed to float through the air, words surrounding us but not really sinking in. "Could this possibly be?" I wondered. Only two months ago we faced the most terrifying news that Terri was facing the deadly disease, the silent killer, and now here we sat receiving this news?
Dr. Kleef systematically reviewed the protocol for Terri's treatment plan and asked him to be at the clinic the next day at 9am. As we shook Dr. Kleef's hand and bid him farewell, there was an aura of magic in the room. It was completely unexplainable, other than me knowing it was just another sign that Terri Mah was going to be okay. He was going to be more than okay. He was going to be healed, and he was going to revolutionize the face of pancreatic cancer and give it hope. What an awe-inspiring, incredible man to whom I was married.

The summary from the official CT, completed on July 20, 2017, in Vienna, read as follows:

There are no enlarged lymph nodes in the axillary, mediastinal or hilar region. There are some fine strips in the dorsobasal region in both lower lobes of the lungs. The structures of the lungs are normal. In the liver there are multiple hypodense lesions which have a ring-shaped uptake of contrast material. The largest are 1.5 cam in size placed in the cranial part of the segment IV., V., and VIII. There are lesions in the dome of the liver in the segment VII and VIII. At the territory of appendix-caecum, there is a mass with a diameter of 1.6cm. It seems to be infiltrating its neighborhood, hard to differentiate from the surrounding fatty tissues- carcinoid? There is a change in size along the pancreas corpus, but there is no real typical tumorous mass.

Terri's Beliefs

We spent the afternoon with the kids and took in the beautiful Schonbrun Palace. Although history and statues did not amuse them for long, they were fascinated by the *cool* floors and, of course, the gift shop. It is so interesting that now when we speak of Austria, they share so many details of the trip with us. It brought to our awareness at a whole new level that sometimes we do not realize how much we pick up on or how our environment and subtle senses truly affects us.

Terri has always been a big believer of this and still is to this day: "You have to do it all!" he always says, meaning you cannot rely on one bucket for true change, healing or growth. We were using energy healing, natural supplements, and beginning our journey with Dr. Kleef at his clinic now.

It all works together, the combination of targeting the body-mind complex in a variety of ways. Terri would confidently stand in the kitchen and look at a carrot, explaining to family and friends, "If I tell this carrot that it is going to cure my cancer, it will." That mindset coupled with fierce determination has led us to this destiny—this blessing that has been given to us. Terri is a warrior, my warrior and now here we stand to share passion with the world. Imagine if we all altered our perceptions, believing that changes in lifestyle and the strength of the mind cause every healthy choice to have that much more impact on our life. What could we all heal from? Cancer? Anxiety? Chronic pain and illness? Are there really any limits to what we can accomplish when we take down the walls, move beyond our ego and access our subconscious mind where the true magic happens?

Like Dr. Christiane Northrup says, "Your beliefs and thoughts are wired into your biology. They become your cells, tissues, and organs. There's no supplement, no diet, no medicine and no exercise regimen that can compare with the power of your thoughts and beliefs."

To truly access our deep beliefs and thoughts, we need to access our subconscious mind. The thing is that our subconscious mind operates as our computer program. When we turn on the computer screen and are browsing on the internet, we do not see what programs are running in the background to make that happen. Our subconscious mind learns from repetition. You can find significant evidence talking about the benefits of going to sleep with repetitive positive statements playing in the background. Terri's story of positively affirming that every healthy choice he makes is going to heal his cancer is building and layering into the subconscious mind. Through repetition, he is reminding the mind at a deep level that every treatment he is doing is working.

Without doubt, there are many moments when fear sinks in for Terri. He would not be human if it didn't. There are instances when he envisions people carrying his coffin down the aisle of the church, or times where he sees in his mind our children standing over him as he lay weak and diminished in a hospice bed. He makes a choice when those fears come in to thank them for coming into awareness, and then tells those thoughts that he chooses to think in a more positive manner. Training the brain, and quieting the ego, he replaces the vision of church with seeing himself walking Vienna down the aisle for her wedding and playing with Nixon's kids. His favourite is seeing us as loving grandparents enjoying babysitting our beautiful grandchildren, and marveling at the wonderful adults our young children have become.

The point is that there is no benefit to beating ourselves up when those thoughts enter our minds. We are human, and fear and darkness are present. However, we all have a choice. Do we rest in that fear or do we choose to move past it? Do we lie dormant and let the fear grab hold, keeping us in our stagnant patterns of life or do we start retraining the brain to a new future? A healthy and incredible future full of endless possibilities, healing and transformation.

The truth is that many of us are faced with dire straits, a tragic blow so harsh that the Universe forces us to change if we want to survive. For the past two and a half years since Terri was diagnosed, we have been learning, changing, and diving deep into every single day. We will continue to do so knowing that these new foundations not only guide our future but the future of our children and generations to come. Changing ourselves to heal and grow is the greatest gift we can ever pass on to our children. It is without doubt a gift that we are both truly proud of.

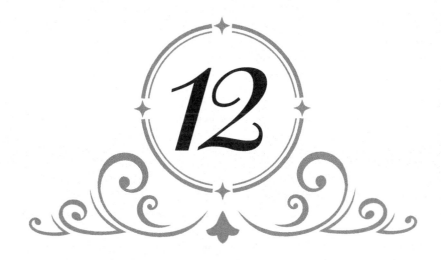

Chapter

10 WAYS TO TALK TO YOUR CANCER

It was the weekend before Terri was going to start treatment in Vienna, and we were out exploring the city. We swung our legs on a park bench and I rested my head on Terri's shoulder as we watched the kids run in and out of the trees at Schonbrun Park. The trees were beautiful, perfectly manicured thirty-foot-tall columns that were a marvel to look at. The kids smiled and explored, gathering rocks and waiting to have our picnic lunch. As we sat there, Terri closed his eyes for a rest, and I thought back to the news Dr. Kleef had given us pertaining to Terri's most recent CT results. I took a deep breath and pondered what factors had led to that success. We were so amazed, so in awe of what he accomplished already, it encouraged us and kept hope in our hearts that he was going to be a survivor. As I watched the kids play, I remembered a conversation that I had with a dear friend.

Sweet Coffee

I loved my coffee with cream and two sugars. Mildly sweet, and ever so smooth, I gave every sip just a second to float on my taste buds and allow my senses to absorb the simple pleasure. On this lovely Saturday morning, I was enjoying a coffee with a friend, and we were discussing Terri's journey. Flashing back to the incredible success he had between the first CT scan showing over twenty-four tumors, and the second one showing that the main pancreatic tumor, and two tumors in his lymph nodes were gone, we were walking through all of the factors that may have contributed. Of course, we will never know exactly which strategy accomplished what, but it was a constant point of speculation.

"One dose of chemo, two IV Vitamin C treatments, and approximately thirty BodyTalk sessions," I reminded Erin.

Erin was new to quantum physics and the journey of understanding the power of the subconscious mind, just as I was. She had taken a couple of classes and had a few BodyTalk sessions herself.

"Hold on," she kindly put a hand up to create a pause in my thought process. "Do not forget all of the extra work you did."

Puzzled, my head tilted to the left trying to remember the details she was referring to. In all honesty, my recollection of the first few months overall was clear, but some of the day to day minute details were overshadowed by shock that took time to dissipate.

"Do you remember the first class that you took?" she prompted me along slowly, a kindred smile warming her kind and beautiful face.

"Why of course," I smiled back. "MindScape. Oh, my goodness, do you remember how I pulled all of Terri's organs out of his body in my mind, and tossed the cancer in the garbage?" I couldn't help but get shivers, as I remembered how Terri had felt the discomfort of the work I was doing in my mind—one of my first eye opening experiences revealing to show us the reality of just how connected we are.

Erin paused a moment, and it became obvious she was waiting for me to arrive at a conclusion I was not getting to quickly enough.

"Yes, of course I remember. Although, let's not forget all of the other healings you performed. You may not have had the BodyTalk foundation in the beginning, but I think it is very important that you do not underestimate the Mindscape healings you were performing on Terri…. And yourself, and the kids." She concluded.

It all came flashing back at once—different visions of various healings that I had performed, every single day. "How could I have forgotten all of this?" I wondered. I took a deep breath, and said, "Thank you so much, Erin. I had completely put these out of my mind as a contributing factor to the second CT. I think because it had become such a habit, an integral part of my day, that it was as commonplace as walking. You know what I mean?" I crinkled up my nose in a childlike way, feeling silly and a bit embarrassed all at the same time.

Erin laid her hand on mine. "Kristie Anne," she calmly stated. "Be kind to yourself. Of course, with everything you have had to handle—researching treatment, organizing travel, running a family, and maintaining a positive attitude for Terri and the sake of your children…" she paused with a sigh. "It makes perfect sense that this may have slipped your mind. I am so glad I was able to remind you of it though. Not only was it very likely a big contributing factor to Terri healing so quickly, but it is also a crucial part of your book." She joked, giving me a little pat on the shoulder.

I took a deep breath and smiled. More memories came flooding back, "Also the *Journey to the Magical Healing Place* CD Terri used," I said so quickly I'm not sure she even understood me.

"Which one was that?" she asked.

"Sylvia Muiznieks's CD, that amazing tool she created. You know, the Advanced BodyTalk Practitioner? For those people who have not taken MindScape yet, it helps walk them through the steps to access their subconscious and create a mini workshop. It is such an incredible tool!"

"Sylvia is always so perceptive at what resources will help move people to the next level," I continued and excitedly started tapping my feet, as I remembered that Terri would use this tool daily as well to perform healings on himself.

We wrapped up the visit and promised to keep in touch. I thanked her for reminding me of the very useful insight. In some ways, it created more questions than answers but through this entire journey neither Terri nor I have needed to pinpoint exactly what did the trick. We didn't feel the pressure or disappointment of never truly understanding what would cause the pancreatic tumor to disappear. To turn it off like a light switch. All that we cared about was to keep doing everything we were doing that our instincts guided us to believe would provide healing, and to have him standing as a whole miracle of a man.

————————◆————————

Give It a Try

For the rest of the day, I could not stop thinking about what some of those healings had looked like. At that point, before we went to Austria, I had only taken MindScape, and did not have any formal BodyTalk training. My understanding of quantum physics was still in the baby stages, but I had one skill that was plenty powerful—determination. I was, and will be, every day determined to guide, love and provide any healing wisdom that God/the Universe allows me access to through my instincts.

Terri and I had very different stories of what the healings we attempted on our own looked like, and that was okay. The point is that we spend time doing them. Time in your subconscious mind can never hurt; it can only offer beneficial insight and opportunity.

Having many conversations about this, we would giggle about some of the silly and nonsensical fun we would have when we were working on Terri's cancer. The point is that you must roll with it. Trust what comes. Work with it, build on it. Imagine you are a child again, and your right brain, full of creativity, is allowing you to paint the most colourful and vivid paintings and create magic. Once I spent time thinking of some of the healings I performed on Terri, so much gratitude came flooding into my heart and soul. As much as they were healings, they were also incredible bonding opportunities that I will cherish forever. Here is a sampling of some of the moments we shared together in my MindScape:

There are a few caveats. Let it be known that before I began a treatment, every single time I invited Terri into my workshop, I shared love with him. I hugged him, held his hand, kissed him, and reminded him that he was the most important man in the world to me and the love of my life. The healing power of love alone is dramatically underrated, and the connection and bond we felt sharing that love every single day on a deep subconscious level was pure magic. In addition, after every experience we had together in MindScape was completed, I would always invite the kids, and Jukie in (our Jack Russell Terrier), and we would all hop into a giant extra-large king bed together to sleep for the night. I would wrap the entire bed with love and hearts and send us floating into the starlit sky to feel peace, warmth, and the infinite possibilities that awaited us in the Universe.

1- I invited Terri into MindScape, and we sat on the couch in my healing room and had a long talk about what fear meant to both of us. For Terri, it meant the thought of not being able to bear intense physical pain, and the fear of abandoning his family. The simple and profound fear of dying too young, with too many incredible lifetime moments and experiences that should be awaiting him—taken from him. For me, it was the fear of losing my husband who was my best friend, my confidant, and my hero. It was the fear of seeing my incredible children who were young, full of life, zest and potential having their hearts ripped out and changing the course of their years ahead. It was the fear of watching the kids have so much hurt and pain in their eyes, just like my dad did when he lost his father at the age of 8. As Terri and I talked, we held hands, we cried, and we swore. We let every emotion run rampant. I went to the cabinet in my healing room and pulled out a fear satchel. Of course, this was all in my imagination, and I was making it up as I went, but I could feel it all so deeply. We took each one of those fears, wrote them down and placed them in the fear satchel. Then we talked about what we should do with them. Burning them seemed cliché and throwing them out seemed insignificant. I instantly knew that we had to face the pain of these fears, and I grabbed Terri's hand and we ran over to the window. This window in my workshop overlooked mountains, beautiful evergreens, and flocks of birds flying in harmony. I encouraged Terri to stand on the ledge of the window with me and reminded him that we were in our minds and could do anything. "Let's jump!" I said excitedly. "As we jump, we can throw the fear satchel away, and those fears will not have the same hold on us. Then let's go and fly with the birds." It took an astronomical amount of convincing, but together we did it. We jumped. We flew. We felt the wind in our hair and tears cascading down our cheeks as we released our fears. What an incredible experience.

2- Before we went to Austria, we knew that the foundations of Terri's treatment would be IV Vitamin C, Hyperthermia, and Immunotherapy. Although I did not know the proper strategies to implement these techniques, this was in my mind and I was treating Terri with love and positivity. I created a beautiful healing corner in my workshop with a Star Wars healing chair, Star Wars posters, and all the Star Wars movies for Terri to watch. Bar none, Terri's favourite series of all time was Star Wars. I created the space feeling like it would be tranquil for him, and I provided doses of the same treatment he would receive in Austria. As taught by Sylvia, your brain does not know the difference between what we do in our physical world, and what we do in our mind—so I knew it could only either do nothing or offer beneficial results. At the end of the day, it gave me the feeling that I was helping and contributing and that was what kept me going and giving me hope, knowing that we were leaving absolutely no stone unturned.

3- Sylvia's instruction also taught us that the belief systems that we form in the first seven years of our life are what unconsciously guide the rest of our life. As we start doing the work to become aware of those belief systems, we can then slowly unlock these and release them. Once released, it is like peeling one tiny layer of paint off our soul and allowing it to shine a little brighter. In my healing area, I had a beautiful saltwater hot tub with a fountain and a sign above that read *Chez Release the Belief.* I remember laughing and loving the name when it came into my awareness. Terri and I would sit in the hot tub together, and like conversation bubbles from a comic book, we would watch tidbits of belief systems float up into the air and dissipate as they popped.

4- One of my favourite healings was when I invited *whichever of Terri's organs* would like to come in, so that we could gain insight and understanding as to what they would like to tell us. When my elevator door opened, there was Jiminy Cricket. No lie. I kept my laughter on the inside, as I welcomed Jiminy into my workshop. Before we were able to begin a conversation, he asked for a tour. I showed him my healing room, office with multiple vision boards and phone, library, and pathways in the forest for walking. Once we finished the tour, he seemed content and asked to sit in the office. I offered to guide him towards my healing room, but he gracefully declined and explained that, at that moment, he was not there for healing but rather to provide insight. He told me that he wanted to sit in my office, so that is where we went. Once I asked a few more questions, I discovered that Jiminy was representing Terri's liver. Reflecting on his character in the movie Pinocchio, I knew that Jiminy was full of wisdom. Jiminy explained that there was lots of work we had to do to heal his liver, but he only wanted to leave us with one piece of advice for right now. He said (which was one of his famous quotes in the movie), "Learn from me. A conscience is that still small voice that people won't listen to. Listen to it," he continued, "And all of this will be okay." Tears streamed down my face. Once again, it was a sign that we were on the right path. Jiminy said Terri's liver was going to come back in many forms along the way, but that he wanted us to clearly remember these words of wisdom from this moment.

5- My primary vision board, or screen of the mind, was a picture of Terri, the kids and I standing outside our house with a banner above our heads saying, *Cancer Free.* On the screen, we were celebrating our happiness that Terri was healed, and you could see the joy on our faces and pure gratitude radiating from our hearts. It was symbolic, but because it stuck to my screen, I knew it was ours. Every time I went into my MindScape, I gave that vision board love and attention. The rule was that when you are in your MindScape, if your vision stays on the screen of your mind, it is meant to be yours.

6- I took a break from inviting Terri into my workshop, and instead I invited his cancer in. I wanted to have a conversation with his cancer. When I opened the elevator, I had no idea what to expect. Out rolled tennis sized black balls. They dodged each other, dancing around my workshop, creating patterns and demonstrating their capabilities of speed and resistance. They wanted me to do the work to try to catch them. I had to chase them all over my workshop, and finally I gathered them together. Once I had them all in my hands, they melded together and turned into a soft black kitten that started whimpering and crying. Of course, since I was in Mindscape and there are no limits, I could have a conversation with this fragile and beautiful kitten. She told me she just wanted to be loved, and she described how the parts of Terri that had grown the cancer did not feel loved and accepted. She went on to explain how the pancreas, whose consciousness in Eastern Medicine and BodyTalk is responsible for *taking in the sweetness of life*, was very sad. Kitty started crying as she elaborated that the cancer had grown because even though on the outside Terri was a positive person, on the inside there was pain, too much worry and self-loathing. The cancer was a wake-up call to change his life, to appreciate every moment, and to welcome every life experience as an opportunity for growth. Once I thanked kitty, aka Terri's cancer, she scampered away, and I felt so much energy and strength. My instincts reiterated that Terri, and all of us, were going to learn from this, and everything was going to turn out A-Okay.

7- Once I learned this information from kitty, there were many days I would invite Terri into my workshop, and I wanted to scan his body for any evidence of cancer. I wanted to infiltrate the cancer with love, strength, and a new perception. Once we had gathered the awareness of why the cancer was there, I wanted to thank it for coming into our life and bringing about this monumental change. How was I going to do this? Well, I was going to use tiny green army men of course! The ones from Toy

Story worked perfectly, the little plastic army men that so many of us played with as children. Terri would lay in my healing room, relaxing and listening to healing frequencies to help realign and reprogram his DNA, and the little army men would go to work. The message was clear, every time they came across one of Terri's tumors, they would deliver this message, "Thank you for bringing awareness to the areas of our life that need change. You did an awesome job! Your promotion is that you get to leave Terri's body. You are free!" Since the physical body and mind are not separate, I wanted to train Terri's subconscious to accept this message that the cancer had done its job and was now free to leave. I repeated this healing strategy daily.

8- Love and gratitude. As we all do, Terri had to learn how to unconditionally love himself on a deep level and feel gratitude for every moment of the day. Love and gratitude are, without doubt, the most powerful healing tools we have within our grasp. There is a healing mirror in my workshop, and when you approach it, you could have a conversation with your reflection. It is an incredibly eye-opening experience. The first time that I spoke with my reflection in my healing mirror and I said, "I love you" to myself, I was taken aback by the response. "No, you don't," my reflection snapped back. "How much of the day are you critical of me- you wish this, you want to change that, you don't like this. If you think you love me, you have a lot of work to do." This was insight that started me on a divine journey of growth and healing as well. Terri would stand in front of the mirror, and although I stood back far enough that I did not need to hear, I could see anger brewing and being released, tears rising, and emotional collapse. It was powerful to watch Terri work through layers of self-misunderstanding for healing and restoration.

9- Sun and warmth. I would invite Terri into MindScape and from all of the research we had done on Austria already, we believed in the healing powers of warmth. We went on an adventure in my workshop and explored different beaches. Rather than just enjoying the sun on a superficial level, we asked its rays to penetrate deep into the areas of the body where Terri's cancer resided and to awaken his immune system to healing.

10- Terri's fear of heights is almost insurmountable for him. If you correlate facing one of your largest fears with realizing the true potential that lies within you, it can be a very freeing experience. One day when Terri entered my workshop, I suggested we go on an adventure. He was hesitant, but willing to trust me. I had created a whole new space outside of my workshop where we could go bungee jumping. It took time, patience, and tears for both of us to feel the strength and be brave enough to take the plunge. When we had both taken turns, we lay on the grass in the field, holding hands and weeping. It was freeing, powerful, and cathartic all at the same time. It felt as though we had released so many belief systems that were holding us back. It is most often not the event itself, but the fear of the event that we need to overcome.

It's not easy for me to share this, to bare to the world the depths of my subconscious, and how I believe those images in my mind could have contributed to Terri beating Stage IV Pancreatic Cancer. It is not something I share lightly, but the overwhelming nudge to write these words was so strong it could not be ignored. If they help even one person, bring hope to one family, then that far outweighs any fear of judgement or ridicule that may turn towards me. There is immense healing potential that lies within all of us.

Chapter

TERRI'S TREATMENT PLAN

Dr. Kleef's diagnostic analysis included the CT, blood work, and an in-depth analysis of the circulating tumor cells in Terri's blood. Upon these foundations, he was able to build a treatment plan that he was confident would be beneficial and have the utmost success.

There was a lot of terminology that was new to us, and a lot we didn't understand. Although we felt confident that we were in the right place and trusted that everything chosen by Dr. Kleef was serving to benefit Terri. Our prayers were strong, and I know that all the prayers and positive wishes from family and friends also helped to strengthen my intuition, to guide us down this path: the healing path Terri needed—for him, for us, for our future.

Terri knew that if he relied deeply on himself, and truly believed our choices would work for his healing, then God's plan would come to fruition. Terri understood that this meant he had to dig deep, beyond the walls and layers of pain and frustration, and reach into that place that held both vulnerability and power; the place where dreams were real and being cancer free was a reality. Based on the quote from Deepak Chopra, Terri believed that:

*You must find the place inside yourself where **nothing is impossible.***

———————◆———————

The Plan

The first test at Dr. Kleef's clinic was the Circulating Tumor Cells *CTC*. A fascinating procedure where Terri's own blood was used to analyze what treatments would be most effective for him personally. The results came back as follows:

Analysis completed on July 18, 2017. Using a modified test system for detection of tumor specific gene expression by qPCR as a measure of the present of CTC. Circulating epithelial cells were enriched by immunomagnetic separation and selected tumor specific genes and a separate housekeeping gene were quantified by qRT-PCR. Based on six positively detected epithelial CTC markers we define the CTC-status as positive.

Following this test, they analyzed the sensitivity of Terri's blood for drug sensitivity. They tested both chemotherapeutic and natural compounds (biologics). Their methodology was as follows: *After enrichment of mononucleated cells by density gradient centrifugation, CD45 depletion and erythrolysis the remaining cells were suspended in cell culture medium and incubated for 5 days with and without the requested compounds.*

Results are summarized in the following tables:

1. Chemotherapeutic Drugs

Compound	Inhibition	Sensitivity
FOLFIRI	59%	++
Everolimus	59%	++
FOLFIRINOX	52%	++
FOLFOX	43%	++
Gemcitabine	38%	+
Sunitinib	35%	+
Oxaliplatin +SN38	34%	+
Fluorouracil	32%	+
Oxaliplatin	26%	+
SN-38	7%	+

2. Natural compounds (biologics)

Vitamin C +aLiponat	79%	++
Artesunate	64%	++
Dichloracetat	63%	++
Digitoxin	51%	++
Cannabidiol	50%	++
Curcumin	31%	+
Taurolidine	25%	+

Rose Bengal	20%	+

These results were astounding to us! We could not believe that there was such an innovative method of testing what treatment would work best on an individualized level, but also that IV Vitamin C, in combination with Alpha-Lipoic acid tested 20% higher than any chemo drug available on the market.

Based on the accumulation of this information, Dr. Kleef formulated a treatment plan. One of the first steps after the diagnostics were completed was for Terri to have a Porta Cath implanted. For infusions and treatments that Terri was going to receive through an IV, a Porta Cath helped to keep things simple, clean and avoid having IV inserted multiple times a week.

Dr. Kleef had us send over Terri's biopsy for review and performed a cardiology evaluation that included both an echocardiogram and stress test.

Here is what one month of Terri's schedule looked like when he was at the clinic:

Monday	Consultation	Dr. Kleef
Monday	Local Hyperthermia with infusion including high dose Vitamin C and alpha-lipoic acid 2X Taurolidine	Synchrotherm
Tuesday	Mild whole-body Hyperthermia Taurolidine	Iratherm 1
Wednesday	Cardiological Workup	Administration

Wednesday	Local Hyperthermia with infusion including high dose Vitamin C and alpha-lipoic acid 2X Taurolidine	Synchrotherm
Thursday	Ipi+Nivo = immune therapy including checkpoint inhibitors Yervoy and Opdivo Massage/Colon Hydrotherapy	Infusion
Friday	Local Hyperthermia with infusion including high dose Vitamin C and alpha-lipoic acid 2X Taurolidine	Synchrotherm
Monday	Local Hyperthermia with infusion including high dose Vitamin C and alpha-lipoic acid 2X Taurolidine	Synchrotherm
Tuesday	2X Taurolidine	Infusion

Wednesday	Long-term whole-body hyperthermia with low dose Endoxan chemotherapy (8 hours in narcosis)	Heckel 1
Thursday	Local Hyperthermia with infusion including high dose Vitamin C and alpha-lipoic acid 2X Taurolidine	Synchrotherm
Friday	2X Taurolidine	Infusion
Friday	Massage/ Colon Hydrotherapy	
Friday	Consultation	Dr. Kleef
Monday	Fever therapy	
Monday	Local Hyperthermia with infusion including high dose Vitamin C and alpha-lipoic acid	Synchrotherm
Tuesday	Fever therapy	
Wednesday	Fever therapy	
Thursday	Fever therapy	
Friday	Fever therapy	

Monday	Local Hyperthermia with infusion including high dose Vitamin C and alpha-lipoic acid 2X Taurolidine	Synchrotherm
Monday	IRD Teeth	Arzt 2
Tuesday	Mild whole-body Hyperthermia 2X Taurolidine	Iratherm 1
Tuesday	Final Consultation	Dr. Kleef
Wednesday	Local Hyperthermia with infusion including high dose Vitamin C and alpha-lipoic acid 2X Taurolidine	Synchrotherm
Thursday	Ipi+Nivo = immune therapy including checkpoint inhibitors Yervoy and Opdivo 2X Taurolidine	Infusion
Friday	Local Hyperthermia with infusion including high dose Vitamin C and alpha-lipoic acid 2X Taurolidine	Synchrotherm

Supplemental to these treatments, Terri was also taking the following:

1. Mistletoe
An herbal medicine that is often used by naturopaths as complimentary to other treatments. It is an immune stimulant derived from mistletoe leaves.

2. Vitamin D
It is common knowledge that most of us do not receive enough Vitamin D from exposure to the sun and supplemental doses are required in order to have a therapeutic effect.

3. Gc-Maf Yogurt
A yogurt that dates to a Japanese scientist Prof. Yamamoto who discovered that there are strains of bacteria in our intestines that benefit from an immune messenger Gc-Maf, or also known as *Vitamin D binding protein.*

4. Low Dose Endoxan
Low dose chemotherapy, oral dose of 300 mg/m2.

5. Ulipristal Acetate
Blocks progesterone. Further explanation in Dr. Kleef's discharge papers.

Throughout most of the treatment plan, Terri felt fantastic. When I asked him about his time at Dr. Kleef's, he reiterated how the clinic was bright, beautiful and everyone was always so friendly. Since Terri was very fortunate not to experience many of the side effects that pancreatic cancer often brings to surface, he appeared healthy, handsome and maintained his smile that would light up the room. Dr. Kleef would affectionately call him *Big Strong Man* every time he would see him.

That's right! That mentality—how he believed everything was working to heal and cure him radiated a light so bright and beautiful from the inside that no one could argue he was anything but a *Big Strong Man*—always has been, always will be. He has just gone on a journey to make that light shine even brighter. In this process we have gone on the journey together as a family and have been transformed. We now view this cancer as our awakening. We may not feel lucky that Terri had to endure this, but we do know it was meant for our best intention. What we aim to do with it is share a beacon of light in this world, to share hope and provide a potential path for those who want to heal.

I found this quote from an unknown author, and it sums up my thoughts perfectly:

If God can turn your night into day, He can turn your burden into blessings.

Nothing could be more powerful, and once we realize that we all have the God-given tools within us to transform ourselves, the sky is the limit. Let me rephrase that—there is no limit, absolutely no limit at all. So, make your goals, heal your pain, and watch your growth transform your life into an inspiring, bountiful reality that you only ever imagined. Just try—there is absolutely nothing to lose (other than a temporarily bruised ego), and absolutely everything to gain. Go get it!

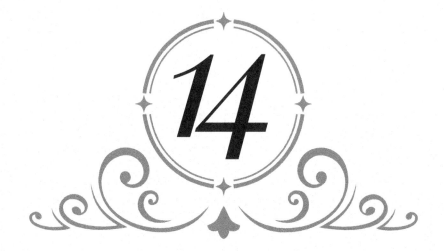

Chapter

LIFE IN VIENNA

Terri would spend his days at Dr. Kleef's, and the kids and I would enjoy exploring the city. Vienna, Austria has been ranked as the number one city in the world to live in for multiple years. Bustling streets full of tourists, the city remains clean, beautiful and very welcoming. Friendliness abounds and is mixed with easy to use transportation and alluring sites. As we settled into routine in Austria, my children grew slightly tired of cathedrals. "Mom, there are only so many stone walls we can think are cool," Nixon would kindly point out.

Intermixing gelato and meringue fingers between museums and churches helped, and one day I tried to captivate their interest by taking them to see the famous Lipazzaner Stallions warm up. Crowded and lined up for what seemed like miles, people of all ages from around the world were gathered to see the famous white horses. Once inside the building, we found a tiny corner upstairs for viewing. The horses were breathtaking; strong, proud and prancing with an elegance and determination I had never witnessed before.

It reminded me so much of Terri, especially of his composure through his diagnosis and starting treatment. He mimicked the strength of the white horses, and the radiant power and determination he carried from within shone like a beautiful aura. You could feel it in his presence, the deep intention to heal mixed with positivity and gratitude for every passing moment.

Of all our adventures, there were two that stood out for the kids. The summer was scorching hot in Austria: temperatures were often above thirty-seven degrees Celsius. What better to do than find the outdoor pools! The first pool we searched out was in the heart of the Schonbrun palace gardens. A beautiful walk along perfectly trimmed hedges, we noticed that visiting the outdoor pools in Vienna was a locals favourite. Eating popsicles and jumping in and out, kept the kids occupied for hours, and every few moments they would run over and whisper in my ear. Let's just say they were unaccustomed to the elderly topless women, or tiny speedos on men. It was very entertaining listening to their commentary.

We would often visit Terri at the clinic during the day as well. There was a tiny juice shop around the corner from Dr. Kleef's, so we would often grab a healthy juice on the way. It was always so calming there, and the nurses and doctors were so kind. They would greet Nixon and Vienna by name, always making sure they felt comfortable and welcome in the clinic. Suzanne, the charge nurse, would ask if the kids wanted to see Terri, and their faces would light up with joy. We would find Terri in one of the rooms, in a comfy recliner, IV pumping him with Vitamin C and quite often the hyperthermia machine connected. Thank goodness for Netflix, as he spent his hours dozing, enjoying shows, and dreaming of his future.

It seemed so incredible to me that this quaint, small floor of a corner building could hold so much power: the ability for one revolutionary thinker, Dr. Ralf Kleef, to welcome patients in from all over the world and offer life-changing results. In addition to his charisma, Dr. Kleef offered a high level of diplomacy. In all our meetings and interactions with him, he remained encouraging without promising results or success. He genuinely cares about all of his patients and makes them all feel incredibly special and valuable. Every choice, decision for treatment, and plan is because he wants to save your life. We all felt that every time we met with him. It was much appreciated as he was always very candid with the information and reviews of Terri's bloodwork and cancer markers. We know what a huge impact Dr. Kleef's treatments had on Terri, and we highly recommend that anyone battling cancer of any kind seek treatment at this clinic. Dr. Kleef offers an inexpensive Skype consultation call before a patient commits to going to Austria.

Terri was apprehensive, at first, to travel out of country for treatment, but here he is now standing strong. The combination of Dr. Kleef's treatment with some of the other methodologies revolutionized our lives. In the process of healing, we have relinquished so much pain, grief and fear. We are people who are here to inspire that the unbeatable can be beaten.

How Fast do you Like to Spin?

There was an entire street, called Stumpergasse, tucked away in Vienna that was full of gluten free restaurants. Nixon, being celiac, sometimes felt dismayed that he could not enjoy traditional schnitzel, so we were on the hunt. Finding this street equated winning the lottery for my children. There was gluten-free pizza, gluten-free schnitzel, delicious appetizers and mouth-watering desserts. Two subway lines away from our apartment, dinner became a full evening adventure.

Once we were out and Terri was feeling well enough to be a tourist, we took the opportunity to find new and exciting parts of the city. Still to this day, our kid's favourite memory of Austria comes from the adventure we embarked upon after gluten free schnitzel one evening.

We had heard about it, we had read about it, but nothing could really prepare us for the experience of attending it: Prater. This place for kids in Austria. Not only an amusement park, but one of the oldest amusement parks in the world. I equate it to the feeling I have watching the movie *BIG:* expansive, beautiful, yet old, rustic and inviting all at the same time.

Comparative to a traditional amusement park experience, there were no lines. I mean none. It was glorious. You could purchase tickets individually at each ride, and the line ups were minimal. Every ride here felt twice as fast and long as what we were used to, and it began to show. Terri can handle the teacups without a problem but the spinning motion on the very similar jetcars lasted way longer; and as he spun around with Vienna, green started to set in on his face.

As we explored the park, went on the traditional swings, and through funny houses, we noticed lights blinking high up in the sky.

"Is that a plane mommy?" Vienna asked. I honestly was not sure, but as we stood and watched we realized the flashing light was the pinnacle of the Drop of Doom tower. We could not believe it! They had a Drop of Doom and Swing Ride that went 150m in the air before it started to spin.

I gulped as I witnessed Nixon jumping up and down and excitedly asking if he could go. Luckily, upon closer inspection he did not meet the age and height requirement. Phew! I was off the hook, for now, anyway, as it's the first place the kids want to go back to when we visit Dr. Kleef again in Austria.

The highlight of the park for us was a ride called Mouse Trap. Imagine a half oval bench that can seat four side by side. Nothing more than a bar on your lap to hold you in, and if you were sitting on the edge and looked over your seat, you would see nothing but ground below you. The track for the car itself was narrow and situated under the middle of the car, so if you were on the edges, like I was, your heart was racing before the ride even began.

"How bad can it be?" I thought, reminding myself that we were not strapped in, so we would not be going upside down and that they let my six-year-old daughter on.
As we went up the track, I let out shrieks of enjoyment. Laughing the entire time, we cruised sharply around the corners and rose higher and higher. Once we reached the top, the seat started spinning rapidly, first one direction and then quickly changing to the other. I used an arm to brace Vienna, just for extra security, but from the mouths of my babes I heard nothing but giggles.

When we reached the bottom, we all wobbled from dizziness for a few steps, and as soon as the kids had their footing, they were back in line to go again.

We ate snacks, laughed, and almost forgot *why* we were in Austria that evening. It was one of the most memorable moments, and even now the kids write articles at school about Prater being their special place.

It always seemed incredible to me how Terri rose to the occasion for our touristy entertainment in Europe. Physically he felt good most days, but the mental exhaustion was draining. Training the mind to believe that you are going to survive is no easy task. His perseverance and optimism, and how he rose to this challenge not only for his benefit, but for our entire family, is beyond admiration. He is my hero.

We all feel this way. Even Vienna, in her own words, and a wonderful eight-year-old Grade three perspective, chose to share how she felt. Her words touch my heart so deeply:

Have you ever had a hero? A hero to me is someone that toughs through hard challenges. Like cancer. My hero is my dad. His name is Terri and he was diagnosed with cancer in his stomach. I felt scared and worried but when he told me that he was going to be okay, I felt better. We travelled far far away to the other side of the world for treatments. Spending the summer in Vienna, Austria was awesome because my mom would take me and my brother Nixon to a huge outdoor pool while daddy was at the clinic. When we were walking around the city it sure was confusing because I heard my name everywhere! After two months our family flew back to Calgary and my dad was much, much better. My hero is my dad because now he helps other people with their cancer to make them feel better by sharing his story. He also makes me lunch, takes me to cheer and even was my soccer coach. He did all of that with cancer and that is why he is my hero. I am so proud and happy to have such a brave and strong dad. My hero is my dad.

What a special gift this story from the heart is to Terri. We are all so blessed to be on this journey of triumph with him, and to share his success with the world.

Chapter

SCOOTER ME SILLY

Weekends off from treatment at Dr. Kleef's meant that Terri was able to spend entire days with us, so the kids were ecstatic! The first order of business, after a few weeks in Austrian summer heat, was to transfer out of our apartment and into a hotel. The lack of air conditioning was not allowing for good sleeps for any of us, and Terri was not accustomed to European apartments with quiet hallways and dim lit stairwells. Transferring to the Marriott, the smile on Terri's face exploded when he saw buckets of tourists floating through the lobby, door men to greet you, and a pool to entertain the kiddos. (They had been enjoying the outdoor pools as well, but the conversations of lack of clothing were becoming a bit repetitive for mom and dad).

When we walked up to the desk to check into our room, we were upgraded to a club floor which included breakfast every morning, and lounge access with appetizers in the evening. As if that was not enough, they presented the kids with a challenge. They had a token Hedge Hog named Swamy, and there was a map and clues for Nixon and Vienna to scavenger hunt their way to finding him in the hotel. It was a perfect way to be welcomed to our new *home* for the next few weeks. It is a memory still near and dear to their hearts, and their stuffed Swamys sit on the nightstand beside their beds.

Once we were settled in the hotel for a few nights, I could see that Terri had relaxed and was enjoying himself. We all enjoyed the beautiful lobby café, where I would sip on a cappuccino and Terri would favor a green tea. The kids would marvel at distinct clothing from all over the world and try to discern which languages tourists were speaking. They would shovel the gluten free eggs benedict into their mouths so fast, I am not sure their tastebuds even had the opportunity to process the flavours. Nonetheless, I believe it to be their second favorite meal of all our time in Europe.

Seeing Terri enjoy European culture, I took the opportunity to propose a couple of trips on the weekends. It was such an incredible blessing that he was feeling so well during treatments, and as Canadians we all appreciate that once you are already in Europe, it is relatively inexpensive to travel around and take in as many experiences as possible.

Kathryn and John were travelling to Austria and Prague for their son's hockey tournament, and it was so amazing to meet up with them. We had become quite close, and Kathryn had been great support for us from the start, and a wonderful sounding board when rough days would wave through.

As we stood in the streets of Vienna, I kicked a rock with my shoe, took a deep breath and said, "He is one in a million, Kathryn," I said, calmly wiping a tear off my cheek. She placed her hand on my shoulder, and with immense love and intent in her eyes replied, "No he isn't, Kristie Anne. He is one in ten billion." It took time for me to process these words, coming from an educated and respected physician. She knew what she was talking about. That comment became the essence and driving force behind this book—those six words will stay with me always. I was forever appreciative.

They had two wonderful boys, James and Liam, and Nixon and Liam played a lot of hockey together. Baby Maya was a new addition to their family, and I enjoyed cuddling her whenever I was given the opportunity.

They met up with us in Vienna and we had a wonderful time eating together, letting the kids swim in the Danube, and strolling around Vienna's core. The sounds of musicians playing outside of the restaurants, while entertainers mesmerized my children with giant bubbles will forever live in my heart. They danced and played, and I took the moment to strategize.

I suggested to Terri that we travel to Prague the following weekend to join our friends there. We would be able to see some of their son James' hockey games and take in the city. Boy I am glad we did, it was such an adventure.

Beautiful Prague

The high-speed train to Prague from Vienna only took four hours. Reaching up to 143 miles per hour, the kids were thrilled for the new experience. Mom and dad snuck in a little nap while the kids gazed out the window and enjoyed token screen time.

I had been to Prague twice before and was looking forward
to sharing it with my family. Such an eclectic city, the culture
resonated through the streets, which were brimming with life.

We checked into our hotel and had a bite to eat. Not surprisingly,
rather than sightseeing the kids wanted to explore the hotel,
go for a swim and enjoy jumping back and forth from one bed
to another in the hotel room. We didn't mind, we knew we
would have the next day to sight see, and the video of Vienna
dancing in the hotel room singing with a bucket on her head was
entertainment enough. Nixon laughed and giggled, trying a version
of his own. I had tears rolling down my face, relishing in the
simplicity of a precious moment of family time. Pillows were flying,
blankets were twisting, and Terri and I had to take up residence on
the floor as the kids transformed the beds into a stage.

Letting go of expectations of what the day *should* look like, I could
have easily been uptight and upset that we were not out exploring
the city. It was a big lesson for me, a time where I realized the
importance of living in the moment and going with the flow.
There is no right and wrong, and I have always struggled to let go
of control. Looking back, I recall the importance of this moment.
How could my agenda possibly be more valuable than the amazing
family evening we had filled with creativity, laughter and cuddles?

Imagine if we all let go of our agendas? The preconceived notions
that things in life must be accomplished a certain way, that
individuals need to behave in a particular manner, or that our
agendas are the only and best way for life to unfold?
Instead, what if we trusted ourselves, God, the Universe, whatever
is your guiding force, that the best plan is being laid out for us. An
anonymous quote says this:

*The Divine Light lives within you, in the sacred temple of your
heart. You have always had the magic within yourself.*

All the love, guidance and power to trust our destiny is within us.
Forbes published an article titled, *Intuition is the Highest Form
of Intelligence.* In the article, they talk about the combination
of research, knowledge and intuition to make the most adept
decisions for our life. How perhaps it will not lead us in the most
successful direction to sit on a stool and do nothing other than

trust our intuition to make decisions for us, but rather to combine our intuition with gathering foundational evidence and then using our intuition to decipher which path is most beneficial for us.

Tying it back to an Albert Einstein quote, the article references the following:

The intuitive mind is a sacred gift and the rational mind is a faithful servant. We have created a society that honors the servant and has forgotten the gift
.

Sitting in the hotel room in Prague, I trusted my intuition that it was the best decision for our family to enjoy a quiet, silly night. We all still remember the feeling of that evening—the love, the fun and the simplicity. It may seem like an insignificant event for which to praise intuition for its guidance, but I often think of intuition as a muscle. The more that you use it and trust it, the more you hear it and can start to believe that it is guiding your path.

Listen to those moments where something simple happens, like walking into a public bathroom and thinking you should not go into the middle stall, and then you say to yourself, "Oh that's a silly thought," and subsequently you walk into the middle bathroom stall and realize there is no toilet paper. Listen to that voice, that rumble in your stomach, or the hairs standing on the back of your neck. Whatever it may be for you, honour it, trust it and lean into it. It will start to open doors to new possibilities and take you on an incredible journey of healing, abundance, and a passion-filled life. I mean, is that not what life is all about? To find that *thing* that lights you up, makes you whole and heals you all at the same time while bringing great abundance and joy? We are all on a journey, and it is no easy quest to start the deep work to get through our shadows and emerge stronger, full of passion and full of love and life. We discovered how truly worth it the reward can be. Do the work, trust your intuition, dig deep into your subconscious mind, find opportunities and treatments that align with your insights. Watch the beauty emerge.

Speedy Fast

In the morning, we awoke when the sun peeked through the cracks of the almost closed curtains in Prague, and within five minutes the kids were ready to go for breakfast. We were not quite so fast, but to Nixon and Vienna hotel breakfast was the absolute best. Delicious options, often including bacon, and the rare treat of having a freshly squeezed glass of juice with their meal.

Once we were finished eating, we went to the town square. Prague is like a fairy tale come to life. Known as the *City of One Hundred Spires*, it is full of culture, and it boasts the home of the oldest cuckoo clock in the world.

We had no plans for the afternoon, so as we looked around the town square, the kids enjoyed the mimes, artists painting portraits—and then something caught their eyes. This young teenager was whipping around on a scooter all through the crowds of people.

"Mom, look at him drive!" Nixon yelled enthusiastically.

"That looks like so much fun, mom!" Vienna echoed Nixon's enthusiasm.

Then, as if planned and in perfect coordination they began jumping up and down together, "Can we go for a ride?" Nixon asked.

They assumed their pouty adorable faces, hands in prayer position, and continued with the bouncing.

"Please? Super-duper please?" they smiled and spoke in unison.

Terri and I looked at each other, and simultaneously shrugging our shoulders agreed. "Let's go see," I said, "Doesn't hurt to ask." Anyone who knows me knows I am always up for driving some fun motorized vehicle around, so I thought it was worth checking out as well.

The young man had stopped in the middle of the square and smiled as we approached him. He clearly noticed that we were on a mission. It was hard to misinterpret the enthusiasm on my bubbly six and eight-year-old's faces.

I introduced myself and waited to see if he spoke English. Sure enough, our instincts had been on par to approach him. He was a young tour guide from England, and the scooters were available for rent. He would be happy to offer a guided tour through the city of Prague on the scooters. There was little hesitation from Team Mah—we were fully on board with this idea. Not only would it allow us to see a lot more of the city since we were only there a couple of days, but it would be such a fun adventure for all of us. We really did want the weekend to be about a break from treatment. Terri and I both had the mentality that years from now we did not want the kids to remember our European vacation as only being about daddy's cancer.

We wove through tiny streets and back alleys that were barely ten feet wide. We all held hands, and the kids thought it was amazing that we could take up the whole street while touching both sides of the buildings. When we arrived at the tiny garage, they had a large sign up offering tours, with a variety of scooters lining the street. The kids immediately chose their favourites based on colour, and Nixon was slightly disappointed that he was not going to be able to drive on his own. As much as I encourage independence in my children and try to be reasonably foot loose and fancy free, there was no way that that was an option.

The afternoon was amazing: out of a movie almost. It was incredibly beneficial that Terri and I are both confident drivers; we drove across bridges amidst city traffic, explored parks, took snack and photo breaks, and stopped to view the famous castle with a view of the city. Our tour guide provided us with interesting information at every vantage point, doing a great job of capturing the attention of my wide-eyed children who were eager to learn, and even more eager to climb back on the scooter and keep driving. The scenery of Prague was breathtaking, but the feeling of the wind in my hair as my children laughed and screeched with excitement is a memory that will not escape my heart. It was one of our most cherished afternoons in Europe, and as it ended the kids thanked us time and again for taking them.

The stories we talked about for days were not the ones of the architecture of the castle, but rather, "Did you see when we almost hit that lady on her bike?" Nixon would laugh and Vienna would chime in, "Or when the brown doggie ran in front of us and mommy had to slam on her brakes?"

After we returned the scooters, we enjoyed an incredible gluten-free lunch at a café right in front of the world-famous cuckoo clock. We finished our gelato as we watched the clock perform its tricks on the hour, and just like it was meant to be, the clock cued us to go and meet our friends to enjoy James' hockey game.

Soothing Sounds

The next morning, we enjoyed breakfast with our friends at the hotel before parting ways for the rest of the summer. They continued their hockey tour, and we took the train back to Vienna so Terri could resume treatment at Dr. Kleef's clinic.

It had been a great weekend, and I often say that I have three favorite sounds that bring warmth to my heart: 1) laughter from my children, 2) the sound of the ocean's waves, and 3) the roar of a powerful engine. I may not have heard or seen the ocean that weekend, but the laughter of my children and driving the scooters with semi-powerful engines (thank goodness not too powerful), left an unforgettable image imprinted in my mind. It was a weekend we would all cherish, and Terri felt rejuvenated and ready to continue treatment. All in all, it was a success. Driving scooters is definitely on our bucket list for our next trip to Europe. Well, Nixon has it on his bucket list to rent a Bugatti and cruise the Autobahn, but that will likely stay on the dream list for a while longer. Perhaps a Ferrari for a couple hours around the city one day, but who knows. I will trust that our trips will lead us to great family time and many more spectacular (and some surprisingly simple) adventures to come. Cancer-free adventures, I might add. After all, this book is about my man being the most incredibly optimistic, ready to try anything, deep-digging, powerhouse of a

Big Strong Man! A man whom will not only be cancer-free but will change the face of Pancreatic Cancer forever.

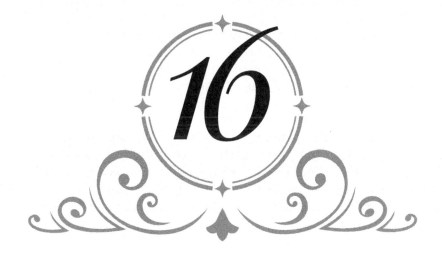

Chapter

CAN SOMEONE SAY GLUTEN-FREE-CROISSANT?

Boarding a plane to head back to Canada mid-way through Terri's treatment was not only a necessity but a wonderful opportunity to see family, friends and our cherished puppy. Terri's brother and beautiful soon-to-be sister-in-law were getting married, and it was an occasion we wouldn't dream of missing.

After the trip we took to Prague, I started talking to Terri about making a special weekend detour on our way home to Canada. Whether it was from advertising in stores, talking at school with friends, or books they had been reading, there was one clear image that my kids correlated with Europe: The Eiffel Tower. Let's stress here, the Eiffel Tower. To them it was more than a monument, it was a pinnacle of perfection in its construction, and I came to realize just how much I wanted the kids to experience it in person.

We wanted to surprise them, so Terri and I planned the trip while they slept. We searched for hotels, booked excursions and flights, and then we even decided to throw icing on the cake: Disneyland Paris! We were more than ecstatic to surprise the kids, and it was not very difficult to change our flight plan back to Canada with a Parisian detour.

Wide-eyed Surprise

Boarding the plane, the kids immediately began to question why it was not as grandiose as the plane we took when we flew to Austria. Coming up with all kinds of unsatisfactory answers, we were able to delay their questions with snacks. We asked them to put on their headsets and have a little screen time to distract them from hearing the flight attendant's announcements about our destination. It seemed to work, and we made it through the flight without further questioning. Once we began to descend, though, it was game over. For little monkeys, they were quite astute, and there was no lack of realization that the flight took what felt like a blink of an eye versus an overnight journey.

We smiled, and Terri calmly stated, "We have a surprise for you." Their eyes were immediately focused on us, and the interrogation began.

"What is it?"

"When do we get it?"

"Is it for both of us?"

"Can we have it now?"

"Is it something we eat?"

"Is it that toy I wanted?"

"Tell us, tell us!"

Their enthusiasm built with each question, and Terri finally explained where we were going. Without hesitation their seatbelts were off, and they were on our laps, hugging us, smiling, and saying, "Thank you." Passengers seated around us could not help but glance over and smile at was clearly a moment of excitement and gratitude.

The next round of questions began, all centered around if there was a pool, where was the hotel, would we see the Eiffel Tower, how many rides are there at Disneyland Paris, is there cotton candy, is Nixon old enough to ride the fast rollercoasters, is it scary at the top of the Eiffel Tower, will the food be good, is there a room big enough for all of us, will we make it back to Canada in time for the wedding, did we pack enough socks and bathing suits, what about Jukie—will she be okay a few more days without us, do we have goggles for the pool, is there a waterslide at the pool, are there some rides that aren't too fast, will we get to meet Goofy, how did you choose the hotel, are we staying at the same hotel or is there one closer to Disneyland, can we wear flip flops to go to the Eiffel Tower, will we be okay because we do not speak French, how will we order food, will we be able to find gluten-free options, oh I wish I could eat a croissant, what else is there to see in Paris, and finally they expressed their appreciation again. We patiently answered all their questions, having to repeat many of the answers as we asked them to let the other finish before answering. Their inquisitive minds are one of the many characteristics we appreciate the most about them.

Lit up Magnificence

Landing in Paris, the kids were anxious to get off of the plane. Bounding with enthusiasm, we had not even experienced any of the city yet and I knew we had made the right decision to come.

It was evening when a taxicab whisked us from the airport to our hotel. The sun had set, and the beautiful lights of Paris lit the streets with a welcoming sense of warmth and anticipation. Since the Eiffel Tower was the highlight of the trip for the kids, we chose a hotel that was within walking distance. Even I did not quite remember just how brilliant it looked be until we stepped out of the taxi.

Stepping out onto the sidewalk, we were focused on unloading our luggage and making sure the kids were safely out of the vehicle. We had arrived on a quiet cul-de-sac and Nixon and Vienna were began jumping up and down, no holds barred, as they spotted the Eiffel Tower beaming in front of them. We were less than two blocks away, and it was spectacular! For me, the Eiffel Tower is even more magnificent at night as the spotlights dance in a rhythmic elegance, captivating the attention of adults, children, and lovers alike.

Their eyes gazed across the Eiffel Tower, looking up and down, up and down, up and down—simultaneously begging to go right to the top instantly. We were explaining that it was much too late, and they barely heard our words as their attention was distracted. There was a beautiful red Lamborghini, one of Nixon's favorite cars, parked on the sidewalk in front of us. Not on the road, not touching the sidewalk, but on the sidewalk. I watched the luggage as Terri moved forward with the kids to investigate and were quick to realize that the Lamborghini had smashed onto the sidewalk. The front of the car was mangled and distorted and wrapped around a light pole that illuminated the front of the hotel. The questions started flying again, "Who was driving? Why would they hit that pole? Were they drunk (amazing how they understood that concept at such a young age)? Are they okay?"

This time, there were not many questions we could answer, all we knew was that this insanely expensive vehicle would cost more to repair than the cost of the vehicles we owned combined. We enjoy life and having nice things but have always said that experiences are worth more than possessions. Right here, on this fine Parisian street, we were proving one such experience. After the excitement of the car wore off, we sat on the bench in front of the hotel, cuddling our kids and enjoying the site of the Eiffel Tower. We promised we would go to the top the next day, and off to bed we went.

***

Hungry Hearts

Our day of touring in Paris was filled with sites of the Louvre, enjoying the double decker bus, French onion soup and a million souvenir shops. We rarely said no when the kids wanted to explore a certain park, stop to enjoy a street musician, or take extra time viewing artwork and statues, questioning why most were of naked people. It had become a family decision that we were waiting for dark to visit the Eiffel Tower, so we meandered around taking in the sites for the day. The real Mona Lisa may have been a highlight for me, but to the kids it was a tiny painting on a very large wall with hundreds of people trying to capture a photo. Maybe we will try that one in another few years when we return!

Our ultimate challenge of the day was to find a meal that Nixon could eat. Vienna and I are gluten intolerant, but Nixon is celiac, and we did not want to risk any cross contamination. Sadly, my fluency in Spanish did not help me, nor my high school French that seemed to be a lifetime ago. It was one of the many moments that I wished I had my best friend Jen in my pocket to be my translator. In many of the smaller cafes we would look at the menus and ask the server if there were any gluten free options, only to be told that many of them included dairy so definitely not. I certainly did not expect everyone to speak perfect English, as we were in their country and doing our best to be entirely respectful. Nixon was just growing increasingly hungry; he was tired of eating fruit that we would bring along and looking desperate for a croissant. It broke my heart to see his face as he glossed over the pastries lined up in shop windows.

Walking back to the hotel, we decided to try the restaurant there.

Call it exhaustion, or intuition guiding us in that direction, but the hotel restaurant was a Godsend. The menu boasted an umpteen amount of gluten free options, Nixon ordered a few favorites and we all shared. Happy and fed, we were back on focus for the evening Eiffel Tower Experience.

Terri decided not to ascend the Eiffel Tower with us, as his fear of heights felt overwhelming at the time. We highly underestimated the number of tourists sharing the same idea as us, and I spent a lengthy time waiting to purchase tickets for the kids and me. In the meantime, Terri took them across the street to the park to buy an overpriced flying toy that held their attention for the hour they would be waiting.

The experience of making it to the top of the Tower with the kids is one I will never forget. Overlooking the city of Paris is spectacular, especially when the sight lines are so dramatically different how from Canada is. We talked about history, how old and delicate some of the buildings are in Paris and watched the dancing lights of the Tower shine on the park around us.

Even though it was an extraordinary experience going to the top with the kids, I am not sure it compares to that first moment they saw the Eiffel Tower when they stepped out of the taxi. That moment resembled fairytales coming to life—something they had only ever heard about or seen in pictures was suddenly right there in front of them, very real and so breathtaking.

We slept so well that night, and even though it was very bright in the room, we let the kids fall asleep with the drapes open. After all, we did choose that hotel for its proximity to the Tower, and it was a once in a lifetime treat for them to fall asleep watching its dancing lights.

———————————————◆———————————————

Speedo City

Morning came much too quickly for me, and I was appreciative of the Nespresso cappuccino machine they had in the room. We packed up and enjoyed another meal in our hotel lobby restaurant before travelling over to our next fairytale adventure in Disneyland

Paris.

The hotel we chose was near Disneyland and had a shuttle that would get us there easily. It had great reviews on the room layout and bunkbeds for kids, and the extraordinary pool that would keep them entertained in the hours when we were not at Disney. Our plan was to let them enjoy the pool as we would be arriving later afternoon, have a great breakfast in the morning, and spend the next couple of days at Disney.

Once we checked in, the kids were very excited to hop in the pool for a swim. Terri had a rest and I took the kids down, and he was going to meet us there later with some gluten-free pizza for dinner. We arrived at the change rooms, and I was informed that Nixon was not allowed to wear his swim trunks in the pool. Entirely puzzled by this, I started looking around and realized there were signs posted. They had a policy against the loose materials on boys' swim trunks. In retrospect, it makes some sense now as the loose material would be easier to catch on a waterslide and tear. As luck would have it, there was a vending machine with skintight Speedo-like shorts (yes, a vending machine!) It took some convincing but once Nixon realized that was the only way for him to enter the pool, he was totally okay with it. He shrugged his shoulders and said, "Okay mom." I took a picture of him in the trunks (luckily there were slightly longer than normal ones available) with the caption *I'm European now* and still to this day we smile and laugh about it.

The pool was fun, completely packed with giggling kids, and they tired out after a couple of hours. We enjoyed pizza and the hotel's arcade room before heading up to the room to bed. We had been to Disney a few times before and knew that a good rest was an absolute must.

A Moment in Time

Heading down for breakfast, the kids were looking forward to the buffet. Something they clearly inherited from their father; a buffet was like winning the lottery. So many options, and often a lot of gluten free ones as well. We were not sure what we would find here though, so we cautioned the kids that it may be an eggs and fruit kind of morning.

It was incredibly busy, so we sat at a table outside in the main foyer. Terri took the kids to explore the meal options, and I asked the server if there were some gluten-free options she could bring us. "Absolutely, of course," she assured me with a genuine smile.

The kids came back with a variety of meats, yogurt, fruit and eggs. Nixon was carrying his plate steadily, but his shoulders were slumped. I smiled at him, trying to lift his spirits. I knew that his sadness meant he had not found any gluten-free toast. As I was telling him that the server was going to bring some options, she walked up with a massive plate for each child. On the plate there was toast, muffins, and.... Drum roll please.... Two types of gluten-free croissants. The look on the kids' faces exploded with an unmatched enthusiasm. They startled the server, and I think they almost wanted to hug her. They devoured them, asked for a second plate (with the intention of packing them for snacks later), and it was one of the few meals for which chose not to enforce any protein or fruit. We just sat back and let them enjoy. Gluten-free croissants—a highlight of our entire European trip! Something so simple filled their hearts as much as it did their bellies.

Hello, Mickey!

Disneyland Paris did not disappoint. It was magical, mystical, and exhilarating all at the same time. Nixon and I rode all the fast and big roller coasters we could, our favorite being the Aerosmith Coaster. Vienna enjoyed all the spinny rides, and Terri and I tag teamed perfectly. He can spin with the best of them, and while my stomach can barely tolerate the motion of a swing set, I thrive on a high-speed roller coaster. Our family favorite was the 3D Ratatouille ride. Completely immersed in the experience of being Ratatouille we dodged and dashed through the kitchen, turning corners to be surprised by rolling tomatoes, and screaming as something fell from a counter and appeared as though it was going to hit us. Vienna and I went twice, enjoying it immensely.

We topped off the day with dinner at the Ratatouille restaurant, surrounded by oversized salt and pepper shakers, wine glasses and cutlery. It was so impressive, we felt like we were the size of a rat. The food was wonderful, and after dinner we collapsed into a well-earned sleep back at our hotel room.

Wrapping up our Parisian adventure the next morning, I watched the kids devour another plate of gluten-free croissants. I was not sure which they enjoyed more and marveled again at the simplicity of children. A simple gluten-free croissant likely rivalled their entire day at Disney. What a lesson to enjoy every moment, every simple pleasure and to never keep tally. It is not a competition of which may have been more meaningful to them. Our story is a compilation of all our memories combined.

We high-fived each other on the way out of hotel, and the kids clung to us with appreciation. Saying *thank you* a plethora of times, Nixon was awkwardly trying to carry his suitcase with his giant mickey hands, and Vienna was skipping as we waited for the shuttle.

On our way to the airport, Terri and I held hands on the shuttle and smiled, no words needed to be spoken. Paris was perfect—it was monumental for the kids, and incredible family time. Boarding the plane back to Canada, we felt confident that the choices we had made thus far were the right ones. Dr. Kleef being the guiding force in bringing us to Europe, Terri had now completed a month of treatment and his results were showing great success. We did not have another CT scan yet to demonstrate anything definitive, but we knew it in our hearts. I always did, and I thank God and my intuition for that insight and strength. I am certainly not saying that all moments were easy or lighthearted, but I always trusted and believed he was and is going to be okay. I am so appreciative for that faith that held strong in my heart.

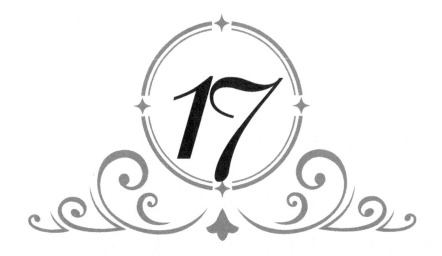

Chapter

HOME SWEET HOME

Home is so much more than a place; it is a feeling: a connection to memories, a safe-haven and full of beautiful dreams. Flying home to Canada reminded me of how blessed we were to call Canada home—an incredible country with beautiful landscapes, safety and freedom. Flying home also reminded me of how Terri and I began our life together—our foundation of love, family, and connection.

Nothing like You

Leaving Spain was the end of an era for me. Many can travel, let loose and find themselves in their younger years after high school. That was not possible for me financially, so a few years after university I had saved enough money, and it all aligned with the Universe to travel. That is a whole other novel in itself—it was one of the most incredible experiences of my life. Having a Dutch passport, I had the choice to stay in Spain for a few more years and make a life for myself or return to Canada.

The choice was clear for me, and I will never forget the words I spoke to Terri. "Hi Ter. I wanted to let you know that I made my decision and have made a plan."

"Okay...." He responded hesitantly.

I took a deep breath, aware of what I was committing to and boldly professed, "I love Spain, but I love you and I am coming home."

Which Way Will We Go?

Two years later Terri and I were discussing our future. There was no doubt that we loved each other, but we often clashed hard. Two incredibly independent people who had lived on their own for years, sometimes I wondered which direction we were going in. I knew in my heart we were meant to be, whether we knew it or not at some moments.

I guess Terri had been contemplating the same ideas and making plans in the background. I had been in Toronto for a job interview and was flying home, arriving around midnight. Texting Terri to let him know that I was en-route, I confirmed I would grab a taxi since it was so late, and that I looked forward to seeing him later.

Sleeping on the plane was never a problem for me, and I felt well-rested when I landed. I was contemplating how the interview had gone, but I had no other thoughts or anticipation running through my mind.

Pulling up to the house I noticed it looked quite dark, and I wondered if Terri was watching tv downstairs. I walked up to the front steps, cautiously as it was icy, and luckily since it was a day trip to Toronto, I did not have a suitcase with me to drag through the snow.

We had recently updated the exterior of Terri's house, painting the trim white and the front door red. It coordinated nicely with the yellow siding and was certainly an improvement over the yellow and brown combination. As I opened the door, I noticed a few spots of paint that needed a bit of touching up.

I took a step inside and called for Terri to let him know I was home. He took a step around the corner (he had clearly been waiting in the living room for me—in the dark), and my jaw completely fell to the floor. I almost collapsed because the sight took my breath away. I could not believe what I was seeing.

Terri was standing there, proud and tall, dressed in a handsome shirt with an elegant grin brightening his face. He approached me cautiously, and as I listened to the whimpers I put my hands out in anticipation. I was not quite sure what was going on, and felt quite shocked, but I was desperate to hold the puppy that Terri was holding in his hands. It was the most perfect, adorable little Jack Russell Terrier I had ever seen.

Tears started pouring down my cheeks, and before I knew it, Terri was down on one knee in front of me.

"Kristie Anne," he spoke calmly and well poised. "We have been on a journey together, through becoming best friends, overcoming distance, and never finding anything more important in the day than talking to each other. We may clash sometimes, but there is one thing I know for certain. You are the most wonderful woman I have ever met, and I would like to spend the rest of my life with you. Would you please marry me, and make me the luckiest man in the world?"

Albeit I did not hear a lot of these words clearly as I was distracted by the adorable puppy in my arms, I screeched, "Yes!" and Terri placed a beautiful diamond ring on my finger. He kissed me, and I felt a warmth that I knew would last forever. Even with ups and downs this was my man, and I knew we were going to be okay. More than okay—we were great and getting better with every moment together.

"Now you have the real Jukie," Terri laughed. I cried even harder as I knew that was the perfect name for her. Over the years, Terri had bought me a few stuffed puppies—one that flipped and bounced for Valentine's Day, another that sat adorably on my shelf. Once I had been at a sales meeting and met an individual whose name was a long version of Jukie. I shortened it, instantly loved the name and told Terri on the phone how amazing it would be to have a puppy named Jukie.

It was a very grand gesture, and I knew that Terri's commitment was sincere. He had never owned a dog growing up, and we joked that having one was baby prep class. When he tells the story, he assures people that there is no way that I could have said no to a ring and a puppy. Then he winks and continues walking on his merry way.

A Glimpse in Time

Our time back in Canada was wonderful: a beautiful wedding celebration, cuddles with Jukie, a hockey camp, and precious time with so many family and friends. It gave Terri a mental break from treatments, he binge watched the entire series of *The Walking Dead,* and the only struggle we faced was the time change.

It was an eye-opening experience reflecting on what home meant to us. When Terri and I got engaged, he officially became my home. Here we were years later with our fabulous children, and it reminded me that whether we were in Canada at our house with the red door, or in Austria for Terri's treatment, we were home if we were together.

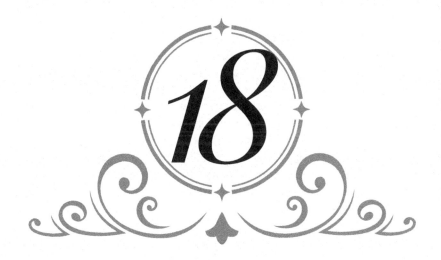

Chapter

FEVER WEEK

Bidding farewell to Terri as the kids and I flew back to Canada was neither easy nor unemotional. Reflecting on the pictures of us saying goodbye, there are so many mixed emotions on our faces. We felt happiness that he was doing so well, sadness to be leaving him, and a bit of guilt as well. Luckily, his incredible mother and sister were flying in to keep him company during the last two weeks of treatment, and most importantly, fever week.

Looking back at those pictures, I remember now how handsome Terri was even when he was bald. The one dose (one dose rather than one round) of full-dose chemo Terri had taken before we began treatment in Austria, had such significant side effects that he lost his hair. Once he began to lose his hair, Terri decided he would let the kids and I have some fun with it. We sat him on a chair in our apartment in Vienna, covered him with towels, and we all took turns with the electric razor. Before we knew it all his hair was gone, but his smile remained just as radiant. I thought that it might be upsetting seeing him with no hair, but it was quite the opposite. The fact that he was losing it from only one dose told me how responsive his body was to treatment, how receptive and open his mind was, and it was just one more reminder that he was going to be okay.

See you Soon

As we left for Canada, Terri and I reminded ourselves that the first month of his treatment had gone so well that we were optimistic the success would continue. It was easy for him to pass the time at the clinic as three time zone changes in ten days messed up all of our schedules; we were often awake in the middle of the night, and Terri would enjoy some pretty glorious naps while he was receiving his infusions at Dr. Kleef's.

We were also very happy that we had taken our trips to Prague and Paris, as after only ten days of being back in Austria together as a family, the kids and I were flying home. We wanted to continue with as much normality as possible meaning that when summer ended the kids and I planned to return home so they could begin on track with the school year, hockey tryouts and the beginning of dance.

Continue the Flow of Positive Thoughts

"Fever is the racetrack for your T-cell race car," Dr. Kleef would always say. We knew how powerful and instrumental in his healing that week would be. Terri went into fever week full of optimism and fortitude. He knew that likely it would be somewhat uncomfortable but believed so strongly in what the results would be, he said he could overcome anything. He reminded me that to him it was no longer a possibility that he would be cancer-free, but rather a 100% certainty in his mind.

Just like this quote from Charles Dickens, Terri continually re-affirmed that he would absolutely do it. He would tolerate fever week. He would be cancer-free. He would be there to meet our grandchildren and he would be there to fulfill his destiny.

He embodied this simple quote:

The most important thing in life is to stop saying "I wish" and start saying "I will." Consider nothing impossible and treat possibilities as probabilities.

There is Nothing like Windows

Fever week was the only time that the treatment was not out-patient. Dr. Kleef had a beautiful clinic in the basement of his house, staffed with doctors and nurses, and decorated with modern décor. Although I did not personally see the rooms, Terri says that the beds were incredibly comfortable, which was crucial for him considering the duration he was required to lie in one. There were large windows with views overlooking Vienna and a beautiful landscape of trees. He often reminds me how those windows saved him from boredom, from focusing on discomfort, and from giving into negative thoughts. He aligned the sun shining through the windows with the benefits of fever week. He felt powerful.

Throughout the entire treatment in Austria, and especially

during fever week, Terri was incredibly appreciative of Dr. Kleef's demeanor. It was so evident that he was not just running a clinic: he was changing lives. Offering inspiration without offering false hope was a fine line, but one that Dr. Kleef knew how to navigate well. His comments were always uplifting, and sometimes it is the simple statements that have the most impact. To this day when Terri comments on how Dr. Kleef referred to him as *Big Strong Man,* he has one of those slow smiles. You know, the kind where the corners of your mouth slowly start to turn up and then before you know it, your vibrational level has increased, and you are absolutely beaming. Maybe, just maybe, those three simple words helped Terri drill into his subconscious that he is a *Big Strong Man.* One capable of anything— including beating Stage IV Pancreatic Cancer.

All Fired Up

The benefits of fever align with both Western and Eastern Medicine. At Dr. Kleef's clinic, fever was induced to help the body become aware of the cancer that was within his body, and activate the immune system to start killing the cancer cells.

Dr. Kleef used Interleukin- 2 to induce the fever, which is a type of cytokine-signaling molecule that is within our immune system. Its function is to regulate the activities of white blood cells that are responsible for immunity within our body. In a simplistic form it helps the body to distinguish between self and non-self.

Working with the same mechanism of action as whole-body hyperthermia and localized hyperthermia, it is another method that intensifies the body's immune response to cancer.

What Lies within the Flame?

Within the Eastern Medicine Realm, it was reinforced how our instincts were spot on to guide us to Dr. Kleef, and for Terri to endure fever week, as the process of visualizing heat and fever mimicked similar healing potentials.

In June 2018, Terri and I had the privilege of coordinating schedules, arranging family to take care of our sweet kiddos, and flying in and out of Vancouver for a one-day seminar led by Dr. Adam McLeod, known to many as The DreamHealer.

By this point, I had taken many BodyTalk classes, and had myself become a Certified BodyTalk practitioner. Sometimes I found it difficult to explain the mechanisms of action and how powerful it could be working on our subconscious mind. I thought this workshop would help for Terri to see and hear other success stories of the power of visualization and the healing potential that lies within us all.

Adam shared his story of the gift of healing he had, and how he taught visualization techniques to share the message that our intentions are influencing our health. Again, reiterating that physical healing goes so much deeper and can be transformed with intention. There are interviews where famous singer, Ronnie Hawkins, shares his own story of pancreatic cancer. After his diagnosis, he received a phone call from Adam who was only a teenager at the time. Adam shared that he knew that Ronnie had pancreatic cancer and believed that he could be of great help to Ronnie. Through energy and intention, Adam worked on Ronnie's cancer. When Ronnie went for his next Cat Scan (CT) the cancer was gone, and there was no trace of it ever being there in the first place. Ronnie continued to lead a healthy life and was awarded the Order of Canada for his contributions over his lifetime.

Throughout the rest of the workshop, Adam taught the audience skills that can be used for our own visualization and healing. The one that resonated with us the most, and that we often share with others for their own healing, is the visualization of utilizing the power of heat and fire. In Adam's words, if you visualize the organ or body part you intend to heal on fire, the heat you are visualizing attracts your body's white blood cells to the area. The white blood cells are the power houses of your immune system, and they are, in fact, what can address the problem you are facing in that area.

This correlates powerfully with Dr. Kleef's fever treatment and shows how the power of the mind can affect our physical body. At the time of fever week, we had not yet learned of this strategy, but were utilizing other similar MindScape techniques.

———————————————————————◆———————————————————————

Family Visits

For all forms of treatment during our time at Dr. Kleef's clinic, Terri had to sign consent forms. For fever week, the form read as follows:

<u>Immunotherapy for cancer patients with low dose check point inhibitor followed by interleukin 2 (IL-2) and Taurolidine</u>

Immunotherapy for cancer patients is experiencing a global renaissance. In particular, the recently approved Checkpoint inhibitors (PDL-1/ PD-1 and CTL4 antibodies) have currently achieved a breakthrough in oncology in indications, previously considered totally incurable. The authorization for malignant melanoma and lung cancer has already been made and approvals for additional indications are expected shortly.

The so-called *off-label* use of these substances according to drug law (AMG) explicitly is permitted, when these substances are already approved for other indications. We have found that the combination of these checkpoint inhibitors with an immunotherapy, which is established worldwide for 30 years showing particularly good results: we combine the aforementioned checkpoint inhibitors with the so-called interleukin 2 therapy (IL-2), a therapy Rosenberg et al published already in the 80 years at NCI (National Cancer Institute) at the NIH in Washington. The substance Proleukine (IL-2) is explicitly approved. Normally, however it is known that an interleukin-2 therapy has severe side effects, so-called *vasculary leak syndrome.* We therefore use IL-2 in much lower dosages and titrate it to an individual therapeutic fever induction in an outpatient setting; additionally, we know that this therapy in the parallel application with Taurolidine, also an internationally approved substance, for port-a-Cath application is known to largely reduce side effects of IL-2. Therefore, during IL-2 therapy patients need to be monitored carefully with clinical monitoring standards. If side effects occur, these are so mild that intensive care medical intervention normally is not required. Loco regional and whole-body hyperthermia often in combination with immune-modulatory low-dose chemotherapy play an important role in this concept.

The safety and tolerability of this method was published in 2006 by the group of Profs. Redmond and at York University in Ireland. A corresponding work was published by Professor Redmond, University College cork, Ireland in 2006 (1).
I consent for the initiation of low-dose checkpoint inhibitor using a combination of ipilimumab and nivolumab. I also consent for the initiation of IL-2 therapy.

1- O'Brien GC, Cahill RA, Bouchier-Hayes DJ, Redmond HP. Co-immunotherapy with interleukin-2 and taurolidine for progressive metastatic melanoma. Ir J Med Sci. 2006 Jan-Mar; 175 (1) 10-4.

The treatment plan for fever week was outlined with the following information, including medication plan:

Medication	Dosing	Frequency
L-Tryptophan	2x1/Day	Evening 2 Capsules
Aurum/strophantus Globuli	3x3/Day	3X3 Capsules/day
Coenzyme Q10	2x1/Day	Morning and evening 1 capsule
GC-Maf Yogurt	100ml/Day	Daily 100ml
Endoxan	1x1/Day	Evening 1 capsule: Start- Evening Day 1 of Fever week
Zofran ftbl 8mg		In case of nausea
Ulipristal		
Berberin		

Important Information:

1- From the beginning of the fever therapy (IL-2 week) it

is obligatory to stay sober. Try to avoid large amounts of meals and/or hard, spicy, fatty foods) starting from 14:00 o'clock, so that the following therapy must not be interrupted by nausea or illness.

2- The medications listed above are to be obtained on time from the pharmacy until the planned fever therapy.

3- Coenzyme Q10 and Gc-Maf are to be picked up at our clinic, so that the fever therapy can be started on the following Monday with all necessary medicines.

4- The admission is 5 days and it is, for security reasons, forbidden to leave the clinic. It is allowed to go into the garden, but not to leave the property. It is acted at your own risk, as dizziness and or nausea can be the consequences. Please, take into account that we have limited accommodations, so only one of your family members (in adult age) is allowed to join you.

5- On Monday (beginning of the fever therapy) you will be picked up by our driver around 5pm and taken to the Clinic Horndlwaldgasse. Please make sure you have enough comfortable clothes with you. Food is also included, so you do not have to worry about the food supply.

6- On Friday (end of the fever therapy), you will be released around 11:00am and can return to your hotel or drive home.

Terri's experience with fever week was overshadowed with optimism. Although at times he found it uncomfortable, he appreciated that he was very well taken care of and provided for in every moment of the day.

On the first day when Terri transferred to the clinic to begin fever week, he started off with a delicious catered supper at 5pm. The way to Terri's heart is through food, so things were off to a very positive start. Throughout the week when we would connect, I would often hear about the enjoyable meals that had been prepared for him.

Terri adhered to a formal schedule for the duration of fever week. Once dining for supper was completed, Terri would put on his pyjamas and crawl into bed. As you could not leave your bed for the duration of the night, he ensured he was well stocked with distractions to pass the time. He had water, snacks, his iPad, and an Android box for the TV.

Once he was infused with Interleukin-2, there were doctors and nurses checking on him every hour, and that remained the protocol for the entire week.

Terri explained how fascinating it was the way in which the body responded to the Interleukin-2, in the same manner, like clockwork, every evening. In the first three hours he would start to get the chills and shivers. He would layer up with extra blankets and was very appreciative of the heated electric blankets that they had on site.

Before he knew it, the chills had passed, and the sweats began— accompanied by nausea and a headache. Terri explained it as a *good old classic flu*. His temperature often peaked between 39-40 degrees Celsius, and though he would never explain the experience as enjoyable, he coins the week as being, *mildly uncomfortable.*

It was difficult to sleep and stay in a relatively stationary position, which made him even more appreciative for the TV-binge-watching. Dr. Kleef prescribed him a natural sleeping pill to help calm his system, and that allowed him to get some undisturbed rest.

Around 8 o'clock in the morning the fever would wear off and Terri could stretch his legs, get some fresh air in the courtyard by the clinic, and enjoy a nice cup of green tea. His mother, Mary, and sister, Caren, would visit daily for laughs, company, and maybe even a card game or two. One of them could have stayed with Terri at the clinic, but because he was responding so well and felt that the TV was enough of a companion for him in the evening, they were able to stay at the hotel together.

Mary would share stories of her adventures around Vienna, and it was no coincidence the first video she felt compelled to show us was similar to a video we took. While cathedrals and museums abound, there was nothing quite as captivating as a grocery cart escalator. The grocery chain, Billa, where we frequently shopped, was two stories, therefore, it was impossible to use a shopping cart; or so you would think. Not at Billa, where they had a shopping cart escalator! Just as it was one of her favorite memories of Vienna, it was one of ours. Of course, the kids perpetually asked if they could ride in the shopping cart down the escalator and laughed for blocks talking about how it was the *coolest thing ever* every time we left the store.

There were four nights of fever therapy, and once completed, Terri was able to fly back home back to us. I will never have words quite big enough that demonstrate my appreciation to Mary and Caren. They dropped everything and were there in a heartbeat to support Terri, and they allowed me to trust and know that even though I was not there, he was in safe and very capable hands.

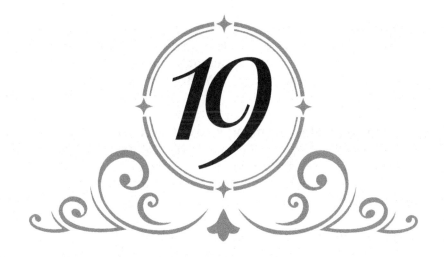

Chapter

THE POWER OF VISUALIZATION

Growing up, most of us have been told to visualize our reality. Dream big, never quit on yourself, and let your imagination guide the course. Whether you had a vision board collage on your bedroom wall that included puppies, NHL trophies or a magnificent garden, I find children are so adept at sharing their dreams. Somehow over the course of growing up, some of those dreams are labelled as unrealistic or silly, and we are conditioned to think life is about the pace of a strong career with the possessions to match.

As MindScape gives us the tools to reinvigorate our visions, it becomes apparent that those childhood dreams must no longer lie dormant. Of course, they may adapt to our current age and situation, but the power of our Vision Board in our subconscious is undeniable.

Sylvia often reiterates the importance of your vision board, aptly referred to as the *screen of the mind* in MindScape, and every time I took the class it helped to improve on technique…. And the more we improve the technique, the faster we can turn our dreams into reality.

This quote from Wayne Dyer supports just that:

The more you see yourself as what you'd like to become,
And act as if what you want is already there,
The more you'll activate those dormant forces,
That will collaborate to transform your dream into reality.

———————————◆———————————

New Layout

I have trusted the screen of my mind in MindScape on multiple occasions and will continually do so. I run multiple screens on an ongoing basis, and implicitly trust the methodology of how it works. In MindScape it is said that if your vision sticks to your screen while you are in your subconscious, then it will be yours. This technique is exclusive to MindScape; however, the strategy is founded on Quantum Physics.

Joe Dispenza reiterates this principle by teaching that if you are in a meditative state (which means you are in your subconscious mind, measured by your brain wave frequencies), beyond space and time in the quantum field, and you connect with an idea or dream, then it must manifest in this reality.

I have seen my vision board bring many things to fruition and have tested it with small tokens and large ideas. The most grandiose way I have physically seen my vision board manifest in physical reality happened one day on a family bike ride.

It was a Sunday afternoon and we really enjoyed family bike rides. We had met up with my brother-in-law Rick and his beautiful girlfriend (now wife) and concluded the bike ride with a picnic. As we bid farewell and were heading back to our house, Terri glanced down Wentworth Terrace and saw an Open House sign. Now, in all honesty, it was not uncommon for us to visit open houses. However, this was different, and I instantly felt it in my heart. I did not know why, did not question it, just simply said yes when Terri asked if I wanted to check it out.

We opened the front door, looking down as we took off our shoes. Quietly saying *hello* to announce our presence as we raised our gaze, it was a good thing we got our words out before our breath was taken away.

We all had an expression that was nothing short of pure awe. Walls of windows, luminescent character, and high ceilings coupled with a magnificent staircase. We were in love. We did not take another step into the house before we announced that we wanted to purchase it. Call it spontaneity, call it trusting our instincts, we knew that it should be our home.

We spent half an hour exploring, kids claiming bedrooms, and inspecting the backyard to strategize where the swing set would fit. We thanked the realtor for patiently answering all of our kids' questions and headed home.

It caught us so off guard, we sat on the couch and Terri and I discussed whether we were serious. I explained that we had a perfectly lovely home full of grace and character, and that we had spent a significant amount renovating it. Terri agreed with me but followed up with one of the most profound and heart wrenching sentences I had ever heard him speak.

He held my hand and in a calm manner, treading carefully, said, "Since we moved to Calgary, we have been in this house. It is a beautiful home, no question—but we have had death and cancer here. I need a fresh start."

It took me aback for a moment, but as I reflected on his words, I realized the impact for me as well. I would often look around the house for dad, remembering the snacks we would share for our tv evenings, or listen for the sound of his oxygen cord dropping as he travelled down the stairs from his bedroom to join us for dinner.

I could not argue with Terri, so just like that we decided to move forward and take the next step. I biked over to grab our realtor and took her back to show her the property. We decided to write an offer. Suddenly, all our dreams for the new home came to a crashing halt.

It was Sunday, and the house had been listed only two days earlier. We learned that it was already conditionally sold and there were at least five people waiting to make offers. Our hearts sank when we asked our realtor Alex Miller, if we had any options. She was always on top of things for us and very keen to be of assistance. She explained that our only chance would be to put in a back-up offer. She was clear in stating that back up offers often did not work, as they often encouraged the other buyers to close regardless of conditions.

Terri and I talked it over and agreed it was our only chance. It took a couple of days to negotiate the terms, and by Tuesday evening of that week, we had the papers signed. It was reinforced to us that we had a minimal chance of the deal coming to fruition.

Hoping and praying was Phase One of my strategy, and Phase Two was the screen in my mind. I took my time going into MindScape, to ensure I was deep in my subconscious. I went through the process of accessing the screen, and I threw a picture of our family celebrating outside the Wentworth Terrace house with a *Sold* sign. It stuck! I could not believe it! Following the rules and trusting the process meant that the Wentworth house was going to be ours.

I told Terri and he shrugged his shoulders, wanting to believe it but knowing that his ego was blocking him from truly believing. I went through the week visiting my screen and giving it love and attention. The picture never wavered and remained consistent.

Friday night the other buyer's deadline was 11pm for their offer to close. At 7pm, we began to get calls and texts from Alex Miller. Updates from the other realtor alluded to the fact that the initial buyer's offer might not go through. We were sitting around the campfire at the lake, and although I could still see the image on my screen, my ego was allowing my nerves to be rattled and fear to settle in.

Then it happened, at exactly 11:03pm, the call that changed our address. The banks needed to hold the original buyer's money for longer as they were moving to Canada from another country. The bank required an extension, but when the buyers requested it from the owner of Wentworth Terrace, they were turned down. Based on our realtor's wisdom, it was written into our agreement that the initial offer could not be extended under any circumstances.

The house was ours! My screen proved to be correct, and my faith in the power of our subconscious mind grew astronomically. I know this story is about a worldly possession and not beating cancer, but it is a clear and strong example of how much we need to trust, and how doing the work can pay off.

Can you imagine if we all took a moment to refocus our lives on the positive, focusing energy on manifesting new destinies instead of being caught up in the day to day stresses of life and living in survival mode?

The truth exists and our power is limitless. A new reality is imminent if we are willing to take the plunge and do the work. Not only is it incredible to watch it unfold before our eyes, but it is invigorating to realize our true power to make our lives what they are meant to be. It is also so much fun. Our ego will try to block us. Rally on, push hard. See past the barriers and knock down the walls. There is nothing but miracles that await on the other side.

Superstar Wisdom

I acknowledge that it can be so difficult in life to know which direction to take, what path is the right one, and whom in life we should trust. The more that we utilize these skills, creating vision boards, reminding ourselves of our true power to manifest our destinies, the more we align with our potential and our new reality. Remembering that the more we trust our instincts, the stronger they become, the more they lead us where we need to go. Eventually, we will stop calling the occurrences in our lives coincidences and realize just how powerful we are.

I will never forget when I attended an Oprah Winfrey speaking engagement. I was ecstatic to hear her words of wisdom and was completely enamored with the grace and presence she had on stage. This was long before I had any knowledge of Quantum Physics or BodyTalk, but I will never forget the one clear message she drove home. She explained that every decision, both business and personal, that she had made in her life needed to be confirmed by her gut. Her instincts were the driving force, her *safety mechanism* for knowing and trusting that she was on the right path. How powerful is that coming for an ultra-mega successful woman? She's a role model to millions.

I will also never forget what Terri said when I returned home and shared the glory of the evening. "You cannot trust your intuition," Terri exclaimed. "You have to make smart decisions!" Oh, how the eye-opening experience we have been through has changed that perception!

Tying into how perception and our instincts can guide and change our reality, Neale Donald Walsch explains it clearly in this quote:

Quantum physics tells us that nothing that is observed is unaffected by the observer. That statement, from science, holds an enormous and powerful insight. It means that everyone sees a different truth, because everyone is creating what they see.

Once our minds are open and we couple this knowledge with

the fact that physical symptoms we may be experiencing are also providing us guidance to what is occurring in our mind, our visualization skills can be strengthened greatly, and we can learn profound insight into ourselves and the destiny we would like to create.

The dreams that we begin to visualize in our minds, especially in our subconscious minds which is infinitely more powerful, can be realized. If you do the work, you reap the rewards. The practice of visualizing, meditating, using BodyTalk and MindScape mean that your dreams can become your reality. Health, opportunity and prosperity, can be yours.

To reinforce the power of visualization, it must be noted that the brain does not know the difference between what you do in your mind and what you accomplish in the physical world. For example, since all information is accessible in your subconscious, you could teach yourself a new sport in MindScape. Let's take tennis as an example. Invite in a tennis pro into your workshop and have them instruct you on the perfect skills. Take a month, or as much time as your instincts tell you, and work on your technique. Then, when you feel compelled, physically take yourself to a tennis court and see how you perform. The results of this type of visualization can be staggering.

It all works together, and it is crucial to honour and understand that the bodymind complex is one unit, meaning that the physical being and mind cannot be separated. Without acknowledging this, we are not realizing our true potential, and the passage from this summarizes it best.

The Holographic Universe written by Michael Talbot in 1991 reads as follows:

According to the holographic model, the mind/body ultimately cannot distinguish the difference between the neural holograms the brain uses to experience reality and the ones it conjures up while imagining reality. Both have a dramatic effect on the human organism, an effect so powerful that it can modulate the immune system, duplicate and/or negate the effects of potent drugs, heal wounds with amazing rapidity, melt tumors, override our genetic programming, and reshape our living flesh in ways that almost defy belief.[1]

And this true story in an excerpt from the same book:

A sixty-one-year-old-man we'll call Frank was diagnosed as having an almost always fatal form of throat cancer and told he had less than a 5 percent chance of surviving. His weight had dropped from 130 to 98 pounds. He was extremely weak, could barely swallow his own saliva, and was having trouble breathing. Indeed, his doctors had debated whether to give him radiation therapy at all, because there was a distinct possibility the treatment would only add to his discomfort without significantly increasing his chances for survival. They decided to proceed anyway.

Then, to Frank's great good fortune, Dr. O. Carl Simonton, a radiation oncologist and medical director of the Cancer Counseling and Research Center in Dallas, Texas, was asked to participate in his treatment. Simonton suggested that Frank himself could influence the course of his own disease. Simonton then taught Frank a number of relaxation and mental-imagery techniques he and his colleagues had developed. From that point on, three times a day, Frank pictured the radiation he received as consisting of millions of tiny bullets of energy bombarding his cells. He also visualized his cancer cells as weaker and more confused than his normal cells, and thus unable to repair the damage they suffered. Then he visualized his body's white blood cells, the soldiers of the immune system, coming in, swarming over the dead and dying cancer cells, and carrying them to his liver and kidneys to be flushed out of his body.

The results were dramatic and far exceeded what usually happened in cases when patients were treated solely with radiation. The radiation treatments worked like magic. Frank experienced almost none of the negative side effects- damage to the skin and mucous membranes- that normally accompanied such therapy. He regained his lost weight and his strength, and in a mere two months all signs of his cancer had vanished. Simonton believes Frank's remarkable recovery was due in large part to his daily regimen of visualization exercises.[2]

---

1 Michael Talbot, *The Holographic Universe*, (New York: HarperCollins Publishers, 1992), 117
2 Michael Talbot, *The Holographic Universe*, (New York: HarperCollins Publishers, 1992), 82-83

It is no coincidence that you are at this point in your life, and that you are reading this book, whether you are facing hardship at this moment or not. Take a moment, and process that truth. There is no assumption whether you are facing hardship at this moment. Something brought you here—to this moment in time, to this opportunity, and to this book. I am not an expert, only a woman sharing a story of the incredible transformation we have experienced in our life. Things were *good* for us. I know in my heart that we would not have gone down this path of learning and growing had we not been thwarted and threatened by imminent death. I had experienced BodyTalk and enjoyed it but did not give it the cadence it deserved. Something always drew me to believing that our intuition was something powerful, but I never really delved into it or acknowledged it.

Now here we are, and our lives have changed dramatically. Some may not recognize it, and that's okay. We are not doing it for others, and that is one of the ultimate lessons. Heal and grow for yourself. In the process, you are healing generational wounds from the past and for the future of your children. Your reality will begin to shift, and obstacles that seemed insurmountable will now appear insignificant. Without doubt, one of the biggest perceptions to shift is that the obstacles are our path. We are not intended to go around them, maneuvering every which way to avoid them. We are intended to go smack-dab through them to mold us into the people we are meant to be.

I guarantee that the more work you do on yourself, and the more you are willing to walk through your own shadows, the more that your entire external environment will change. As it was said above, we are all creating our own realities. If we were to climb into someone else's body, the physical world would appear entirely different. That is the power we have—to change our realities. The power to heal. To opportunity to grow. The ability be prosperous.

To enjoy the beauty of our time on Earth. To deepen our connection with God and the Universe. To smile because we are so deeply in love with life. To experience gratitude daily so deep that our hearts feel as though they are going to explode. To be cancer free. To be headache free. To be high-cholesterol level free. The list is endless, and the potentials are equally as boundless.

You are here for a reason. Calm that ego and take the plunge. Dive deep and watch your new reality unfold. You have absolutely nothing to lose and absolutely everything to gain. I will not promise that walking through the shadows is always easy, but I will promise that it is one-hundred-percent worth it. The new destiny is nothing short of a vision of beauty.

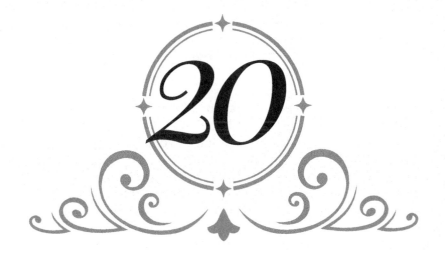

Chapter

BODYTALK BREAKTHROUGHS

BodyTalk is an incredible modality of healing that can be of benefit to anyone. Rather than looking at the body as independent parts, the system takes into consideration the entire bodymind complex for healing. What this means is that BodyTalk addresses the whole person and their whole story. The physical, emotional, mental, spiritual, and environmental are all taken into consideration.

On the International BodyTalk Association Website, it is defined as follows:

BodyTalk is a simple and effective holistic therapy that allows your body's energy systems to be re-synchronized so they can operate as nature intended.

Through all the advanced classes I took from Sylvia, I find it easiest to explain this way—your entire body holds the consciousness and energy of all its parts. For example, if your ankle is hurting, the symptom of it being from your ankle can be treated, however the original cause for your ankle pain may not originate from your ankle. It may, instead be the memory of a childhood trauma that your body has stored in your ankle, and the physical pain in the ankle is your body's way of expressing its unwillingness to be adaptable or take a step forward. This is only one of a million examples it could be.

It takes a shift in mindset, to understand how interconnected not only the physical body is, but the body and mind are together. Our subconscious minds operate as our computer, constantly running and functioning in the background. When it gets overloaded, it can cause malfunctions within our BodyMind complex. How does it get overloaded? Here are some examples (certainly not an all-inclusive list) of how overload in our subconscious can occur:

- ❖ Unprocessed emotions
- ❖ Trauma endured in life
- ❖ Generational factors
- ❖ Physical injury
- ❖ High levels of stress

We operate at full-on capacity in our day and age, which can take a physical and mental toll on our bodies. When we operate in survival mode, just getting through the day, there is so much that we do not acknowledge, process and release. It then remains stored in our body and if continually unaddressed can begin to appear as physical symptoms. Those symptoms are intended to bring awareness and captivate our attention to look deeper.

This is exactly what happened to Terri. My husband is an incredibly positive, salt-of-the-earth man who viewed life as an opportunity for fun and experiences. However, over the years you could see that he was being weighed down with emotion. His drive to take care of himself was lacking, and he now admits that he was a closet worrier who appeared to be positive in his conscious mind, which was only a tiny five percent of his mind. The rest was running thoughts of worry and stress. My point is this-life always presents challenges and obstacles that we need to work through. If we consciously speak and think that all is good, it is a step in the right direction, but we are literally not in the right frame of mind to propel true change in our life. We need to get into our subconscious mind, which is the bottom of the iceberg. It encompasses over ninety-five percent of our mind and is the only place we can impact true change. MindScape, BodyTalk, and meditation are examples of strategies people employ to do this.

You see, once Terri was diagnosed, he began to open-up, explaining to me how much he worried daily. Worrying about whether the kids would be hit by a car as they biked to school, worrying if losing a sports event would be too damaging for them, or worrying if we would be financially okay during a period of recession. The worries continued into wondering if I was going to find another career position I really liked, worrying about his parents and if they were okay, worrying about if we made the right decision relocating to Calgary, worrying if the kids were going to like their new school and fit in, worrying about if he could be successful again in his new territory for work…. The list went on and on. I was honestly shocked, yet appreciative, when he started to share all these concerns with me. Can you imagine, though, if these are the worries that come to him off the top of his conscious mind what the deep layers of these are in the subconscious?

This is where BodyTalk came in. Essentially, BodyTalk is based on the belief that the body knows how and is fully capable of healing itself. It has the *innate ability and wisdom* to heal itself. In my opinion, one of the factors most intriguing about BodyTalk is the tie to Eastern Medicine and how each of our organs and body parts have a consciousness to them. For example, your lungs serve their function in Western Medicine to help you breathe. There are many, but one of the consciousnesses of your lungs in Eastern Medicine is grief.

Recalling the story of my dad passing away from lung cancer— there were other contributing factors, as he was a smoker, but my instincts tell me the catalyst of the lung cancer was grief. Before he was diagnosed, he had recently become engaged and was madly in love. It went sideways, and shortly afterwards he ended up with a massive heartache. He was grieving the loss of his fiancé, and it quite possibly manifested itself as lung cancer.

Tying it back to Terri's diagnosis, in Eastern Medicine the consciousness of the pancreas is *taking in the sweetness of life.* The opposite of that is worry. So, when the pancreas cannot keep up with processing copious amounts of worry, the bodymind complex is out of balance.

These stories are used to provide insight as to what may occur in the bodymind complex, but BodyTalk never diagnoses or prescribes. It simply taps into the energetic circuits of the body using simple muscle testing that has been around for hundreds of years. Different techniques are used for the body to adopt the changes being made, as your innate ability brings to the surface what is a priority for your body.

BodyTalk was founded by Dr. John Veltheim and is now taught and practiced all over the world. Dr. Veltheim is an expert in Chinese medicine, acupuncture, chiropractic and naturopathy. He blended these different strategies to create BodyTalk. Once you tap in the formulas that have arisen during the session, the body downloads and adopts the changes. It's different than a computer downloading a program. Sylvia has worked closely with Dr. Veltheim to develop the methodologies implemented in the Advanced Modules. Aside from learning the material in her classes, Terri and I both have had many personal BodyTalk sessions from her, and her abilities to tap into the root cause of underlying dis-ease (with incredible tact and grace) is phenomenal.

Speaking as a Certified BodyTalk Practitioner, the training to learn this incredible system is not only intriguing, but it's amazingly fun and healing in the process. During my first four-day BodyTalk training class with the talented Allison Bachmeier, I felt so many shifts and my mind felt clearer and more focused than it had in years. I joked that it felt like the equivalent of having fifteen chiropractic sessions, ten counselling sessions, and a few physio appointments as well. It was a path that once started, I knew I would never look back. I have taken extensive classes, and although I am not practicing full-time, I still provide numerous sessions and ensure that all members of my family are receiving sessions on a monthly basis.

The most profound awareness for me is this—we are not taught as practitioners to decide what *seems* to be best for the client. There are extensively detailed protocol charts we follow, however, we are not making decisions. We are taught how to tune in and listen to the innate wisdom that the client's body and mind are providing. They are doing the healing; they are bringing to the surface what needs acknowledgement, and we are simply witnesses to walk them down the path and provide feedback as to the awareness they are experiencing. Every single practitioner, including Dr. Veltheim himself, are witnesses to miraculous stories of transformation. It all ties back to the whole premise of this book—trust yourself and do the work!

A Personal Session

Circling back to the BodyTalk treatments Terri had before we travelled to Austria, Terri may not have understood the meaning of some of the formulas and that was okay. He trusted the process and found the session recordings from my friend very comforting. That is another amazing component of BodyTalk—once you observe what your higher self brings up, it has come into your awareness and is released. There is nothing more that needs to be done. We must trust the process. Additionally, it is irrelevant whether you understand the content of a BodyTalk session because as your body and its innate wisdom have done the work bringing it to awareness. What a phenomenal method to provide healing, growth, and insight into our true selves.

To provide a glimpse into some of Terri's sessions, one of

the first formulas, of the first session he gave himself and his body, "Permission for my body to respond to BodyTalk." Subsequently, he gave his mind, "Permission for my mind to be open to BodyTalk." This was coupled with releasing a measure of intolerance to fear that was being stored in the pancreas, while reinforcing a belief system in his heart of self-love that, "It is safe to love myself." Although I will not outline the entire session, I will say that there were also Cortices in the formula and Hydration of the liver. Cortices is the foundation of BodyTalk, used to balance the left and right side of the brain to work more effectively together. It is said that often the two sides of the brain spend time competing and conflicting, so Cortices assists them in functioning as a team. Hydration of an organ or body part is hydrating it with water and with joy.

For almost one year my friend performed a minimum of three BodyTalk sessions a week on Terri. Their significant effect on his treatment and healing still amazes us to this day. When we were sitting in Dr. Kleef's office for the initial visit after his CT in Austria, and he explained that Terri was in partial remission, we could not believe our ears.

BodyTalk is a complimentary tool that can be combined with any other type of treatment in either Western or Eastern medicine. It is a gentle approach that offers new insight into the origin of the obstacle you may be overcoming, and as you heal and grow, it will amaze you the degree to which your mind becomes responsive as well.

I welcome you to explore the International BodyTalk Association website to find a practitioner near you. The website also includes a plethora of information and interviews with Dr. Veltheim, during which he provides demonstration sessions. We are lucky to have the talented Sylvia Muiznieks right here in Alberta. Additionally, there are numerous other certified practitioners in the province, country, and across the globe.

The world is our oyster—thank your ego for protecting you along the way, and welcome openness of new modalities to grow, heal and take down those protective barriers that may be standing in the way of your true destiny. The path may be difficult at times, but that only makes coming out the other side that much more rewarding. Don't wish for change; do the work and make it happen. There are so many support systems out there, including the BodyTalk method, to help guide you along the way. It just takes reaching out. You can do it!

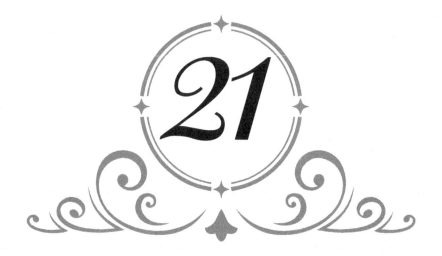

Chapter

DR. KLEEF'S DISCHARGE PAPERS

The two months that Terri spent in Austria were more impressive than we could have imagined: the quality of the treatments and the etiquette of the staff at the clinic were only unparalleled by Dr. Kleef himself. We are so grateful for the opportunity to meet such a rare individual who can combine passion, knowledge, and offer life-changing treatment in a safe and welcoming environment.

Since the time that Terri was in Austria, we have continually recommended Dr. Kleef to other individuals facing cancer. We will continue to do so, as we had fabulous success combining Dr. Kleef's treatments with other methodologies including MindScape and BodyTalk.

I knew that it would be of great interest to those with a clinical curiosity to have the opportunity to review the treatments that were included in Terri's time at the clinic. Please see below Terri's official discharge papers: they have composed by Dr. Kleef himself who has given us explicit permission to share.

Clinical Discharge Letter

September 22, 2017

We summarize the diagnostic procedures and therapies we performed for Terri Mah during the treatment cycle in Vienna:

Diagnosis: Pancreatic cancer, liver metastases, peritoneal carcinosis.

Duration of stay in our outpatient department:
18th July 2017- 15th September 2017

Medical History

First diagnosis 05/2017 the patient underwent histological confirmation of primary inoperable adenocarcinoma of the pancreas with disseminated liver metastasis and a single large peritoneal deposit close to the caecum. There was small volume ascites.

The patient was offered 4 options of first line palliative therapy:
1- W & W
2- Gemcitabine mono
3- Gemcitabine/Abraxane (protein bound paclitaxel)
4- Folfirinox

On July 2nd, 2017 received the 1st line CHT with gemcitabine-Abraxane.

CA: Karnofsky Index 90%; the patient experienced mild left upper abdominal discomfort which started around 9 months ago and realized persistent similar pain for 2 months VAS 2-3. The patient does not need any pain medication currently.

Physical examination: Skin: clear, no jaundice, no peripheral edema. One left axillary 1cm palpable enlarged lymph node. Tongue is wet, clear. Chest: lungs are clear, no SOB; Heart: regular, normal heart sounds, no murmurs. HR; 64/min. Abdomen: soft, liver is hardly palpable. Stool is regular, sometimes loose, but rather shaped, well colored. Extremities and joints are free in motion, muscle tone is normal. No signs of neurological defect.

Social history: The patient is a native Canadian with Chinese origin, married and has 2 children aged 5 and 7, works as sales rep in a generic pharmaceutical company. He is attended by his wife and 2 children.

Plan:
1- LABD with cytokine profile, TM CEA, CA 19-9, Thymidinkinase
2- CTC/TCA
3- IRD Teeth
4- CT Thorax/Abdomen
5- Porta-Cath Implantation, possibly second biopsy
6- MDT Oncobrain
7- Shipment of Paraffin material from Canada for Pantherchip for Laboratory Professor Bojar, Germany
8- Cardiology evaluation including echocardiogram and stress test
9- THY li Abdomen Sycrotherm/Andromedic with INSA
10- MH
11- LD CI

12- LD-WBH with low dose Endoxan 300 mg/m2
13- IL-2
14- Gc-Maf Yogurt
15- Ulipristal Acetate

Treatments

1. Local RF Hyperthermia/High dose Vitamin C/Alpha Lipoic Acid

Loco-regional radiofrequency deep hyperthermia 13.56 MHz was administrated 14 times to the abdominal region in combination 11 times with high dose (0.5 g/kg) Vitamin C and alpha lipoic acid (INSA/ALA).

Number	dd.mm. yyyy	Description	Code
14	18.07.2017-15.09.2017	Local RF (Radio Frequency) Hyperthermia 13.56 MHz, max 400W	THY
11	18.07.2017-15.09.2017	High Dose Vitamin C (0.5 mg/kg) and Alpha Lipoic Acid	INSA

2. Checkpoint inhibitor therapy in combination with Taurolidine (1)

The patient underwent 2 cycle of weekly low-dose checkpoint inhibitor therapy with PD1/PDL-1 inhibition with nivolumab (0.5 mg/kg) and CTL-4 inhibition with ipilimumab (0.3 mg/kg) over three weeks which was followed by:
(NOTE: due to mildly elevated liver enzymes (autoimmune hepatitis could be side effect of the immunotherapy) following the second dose of immunotherapy we ceased the delivery of third dose.)

Week	dd.mm. yyyy	Ipilimumab	Nivolumab	Taurolidine	Code
1.1	01.08.2017	18.9 mg	31.5 mg	3 x 250ml	YERV
1.2	24.08.2017	12.2 mg	18.3 mg	3 x 250 ml	YERV

Immune modulating chemotherapy in combination with whole body hyperthermia

Fever- range whole body hyperthermia (FR-LD-WBH) in combination with low-dose cyclophosphamide 300mg/ m2 to prevent TReg cell (CD4 CD25 CD127 in % of T4) induction. During the FR-LD-WBH the patient was monitored with intensive care standards, and slightly sedated with a combination of midazolam and Propofol, followed by:

Number	dd.mm. yyyy	Chemotherapy	Hyperthermia	Code
4	19.07.2017., 03.08.2017., 22.08.2017., 12.09.2017		Mild whole-body hyper-thermia	MH
1	30.08.2017	Cyclophospha-mide 300mg/m2- TD: 609mg	Long-term whole-body hyperthermia	LZGK

Moderate dose Interleukin-2 (IL-2) therapy under Taurolidine protection

5 days interleukin-2 (IL-2) (decrescendo regime) therapy under Taurolidine protection. IL-2 has been developed in the late 80s by the group of Steven Rosenberg at NCI in Washington and has been shown to be one of the most powerful activators of T-cell mediated immunity. Because of the potential danger including capillary leak syndrome and critical patient management in the intensive care we combine IL-2 with Taurolidine in an off-label use. Taurolidine is licensed for the intravenous blockage of Port-a-Cath systems to prevent infections. Interestingly, it has been shown that Taurolidine can greatly prevent the side effect of IL-2. The patient 2 times underwent these 5 days monitoring undergoing IL-2 therapy combined with Taurolidine starting on the following dates:

Number	dd.mm. yyyy	Description	Code
1	04.09.2017- 08.09.2017	Proleukin Therapy	IO

3. **Chemotherapy**

According to the tumor chemosensitivity assay we delivered metronomic low dose chemotherapy on the following dates:

Number	dd.mm. yyyy	Chemotherapy	Code
3	02.08.2017., 25.08.2017., 01.09.2017.	Gemcitabine 500mg/ m2- TD: 585 mg, Gemcitabine 500mg/ m2- TD: 5 Gemcitabine 500mg/m2- TD: 585 mg, 85 mg,	CHT

4. Ulipristal acetate

Ulipristal acetate can modulate and activate Natural killer cells which belong to the so-called innate immune system and play an important role in preventing and fighting cancer. Very often these cells of our innate and adapted immune system are blocked by complex immune suppressive mechanisms mediated directly in the tumor micro-environment. Amongst many suppressive cytokines and malignant inflammatory parameters one factor is "progesterone induced blocking factor" (PIBF).

American Cancer researchers have found out that "mifepristone" (normally used in birth control as Mifegyne) is inhibiting this intracytoplasmic immunomodulatory protein known as PIBF. This in turn allows the cellular immune cells (especially natural killer (NK) cells) to attack the rapidly growing tumor cells. Since mifepristone is extremely expensive and only restricted for the use in birth control clinics, we found out that a nearly identical preparation called "Ulipristal acetate" (UP) has the same effects and can be prescribed by us in an "off-label" use. The substance is marketed in Europe as "Ella One" and is registered for the treatment of uterine fibroid(s).

One times daily Ulipristal acetate 30mg together with 1 capsule of Berberin 400mg ideally with a glass of grapefruit juice in the morning; (the science behind this: Berberin and grapefruit juice slowdown the enzymatic degrading of UP in the liver leading to longer half-time in the body).

List of Current Medication

Drug Name	Dosage
Tbl. Celebrex 200mg	1-0-0-0
Tbl. Endoxan 50mg	1-0-1-0
Caps. NN Coenzyme Q10	1-0-1-0
Tbl. Ulipristal/Berberin	1-0-0-0
Caps. L-Tryptophan	1-0-1-0
Cannexol 10%	5 to 10 drops 3 times daily

Epicrisis

The patient was admitted to our outpatient care with the diagnosis of metastatic pancreatic cancer. He underwent our complex immune-chemo-thermotherapy cycle. He tolerated all the therapeutic activities relatively well. Two weeks following the second dose of immunotherapy in his laboratory values a mild elevation of liver enzymes were seen. Thus- since the CI therapy can be the promoter for autoimmune hepatitis- the third dose of immunotherapy was cancelled. The delivery of the missing dose will be possible, following the return of the liver enzymes to normal range.

Following our treatment circle his TM-CEA dropped to the normal range of 0.7 ng/ml from the elevated value of 3.9 ng/ml measured on 21.08.2017.
At the time of discharge his condition is stable, his physical activity is appropriate to his lifestyle, he is in good mood and emotional state. Even his liver enzymes already started to normalize, but still elevated (14.09.2017). As they will return to the normal, we're waiting for the return of the patient.

Further recommendations and follow up plan:

1- Gemcitabine 500 mg/m2 Day: 1, 8, 15, repeat every 28 days
2- High dose Vitamin C -0.5mg/kg plus alpha lipoic acid 600 mg in a separate infusion on the chemotherapy date

We recommend recheck important markers in the blood, e.g. WBC, HGB, PLT, liver and kidney functions, blood sugar weekly and thyroid function, tumor markers bi-weekly/monthly. Further we recommend repeating the CT-scan within 2-3 months following our treatment cycle. We kindly advise to share the latest results of scan and bloodwork with us via email. The necessity of the second treatment cycle, possible on early winter season of 2017, will be assessed on the base of newest results.

My whole team and myself send our very best wishes to this dear patient.

Dr. Ralf Kleef

References:
1- This is an off-label use of the active substance Taurolidine, of which extensive studies as neoangiogenesis inhibitors and cytostatic drub were published. Taurolidine is a redox-oriented, broad-spectrum cancer agent with a dual mechanism of action in surgical oncology. It induced ROSH mediated mechanisms of oxidative stress in cancer cells (apoptosis/programmed cell death) and Autophagy and prevents neovascularization by suppressing VEGF production and VEGF induced lumen formation and down modulates chronically elevated proinflammatory cytokines. A venous Port-a-Cath is required for the system administration of Taurolidine.
2- Further relevant references of Taurolidine in cancer therapy:
    1. Neary P et al: the evolving role of taurolidine in cancer therapy. Ann Surg Oncol. 2010 April 17(4); 1135-43
    2. O'Brien GC et al: Co-immunotherapy with interleukin-2 and taurolidine for progressive metastatic melanoma. Ir J Med Sci 2006 Jan-Mar; 175(1): 10-4
    3. Braumann C et al: Taurolidine reduces the tumor stimulating cytokine interleukin-1beta in patients

with resectable gastrointestinal cancer; a multicenter prospective randomized trial. World J Surg Onc. 2009 Mar 23; 7:32. Doi: 10.1186/1477-7819-7-32

4. Marley K et al: The effects of taurolidine alone and in combination with doxorubicin or carboplatin in canine osteosarcoma in vitro. BMC Vet Res. 2013 Jan 18; 9:15. Doi: 10.1186/1746-6148-9-15

5. Harati K et al: TRAIL and taurolidine enhance the anticancer activity of doxorubicin, trabectedin and mafosfamide in HT1080 human fibrosarcoma cells. Anticancer Res. 2012 Jul; 32 (7): 2967-84

6. Chromik AM et al: Gene expression analysis of cell death induction by taurolidine in different malignant cell lines. BMS Cancer. 2010 Oct 30; 10:595. Doi; 10.1186/1471-2407-10-595

7. Stendel R et al: The antibacterial substance taurolidine exhibits anti-neoplastic action based on a mixed type of programmed cell death. Autophagy. 2009 Feb; 5(2): 194-210. Epub 2009 Feb 13.

8. Jacobi CA et al; Ta277-86urolidine- a new drug with anti-tumor and anti-angio-genic effects. Anticancer Drugs. 2005 Oct; 16 (9) 17-21

9. Matuschek C et al: Methylated APC and GSTP1 genes in serum DNA correlate with the presence of circulating blood tumor cells and are associated with a more aggressive and advanced breast cancer disease. Eur J Med Res. 2010; 15: 277-86

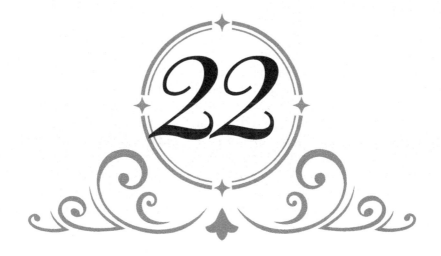

Chapter

22

MY WIFE, MY HEALER

Watching the sun set and rise as Terri flew back to Canada, he counted his blessings. He told me that he drifted off to sleep making a list in his mind of all that he had incredible gratitude for in his life. Without doubt, the obvious items were there— his wife and children, family and health. He felt gratitude for how successful the treatment was, and the generosity from the community allowing us to travel to Austria in the first place. Between a Go Fund Me Page, and the fundraising evening in Saskatoon, we had raised over $100,000. Couple that with family donations that were beyond generous gave us an incredible start to funding the improvement of Terri's overall health.

The gratitude Terri was experiencing went beyond these monumental items and extended to some of the finer and more minute details of life. Having a roof over our heads, food on the table, and the ability to fund our kids' activities thanks to a career that he loved, did in fact make us incredibly blessed and more fortunate than much of the world's population. We always recognize that, give back when we can, and encourage others to do the same. It was not so many years ago that we funded the building of a school in Nicaragua, and seeing the picture of the children outside of the school beaming allows us to remind our own kids of their incredible good fortune to be living where we live and receiving an excellent education.

Another aspect of his gratitude was genuine appreciation for the company he worked for over the last decade. Terri had been an employee of Apotex for more than ten years and at this point had it in his heart to spend the rest of his career with them. He was incredibly loyal to them, which is why he was willing to relocate from Saskatoon, Saskatchewan to Calgary, Alberta when it was required. He is a sales representative for the company, and a born salesman he is. Terri lights up a room when he enters and has formed great partnerships with his customers that have brought him profound success in his years with Apotex. Terri's manager and colleagues were a fundamental part of the fundraising evening held for Terri, and it was greatly appreciated.

Apotex has been incredibly generous to Terri, providing him the time off he needed for treatment and giving him the options available within the company's HR portfolio. Encouragement and support rolled in continuously from colleagues, directors and even the founder of Apotex, Barry Sherman who passed along best wishes. That is incredible for a company with over 10,000 employees!

Once Terri returned from Austria, he took time to recover from jetlag, allow the treatments from Dr. Kleef's clinic to take effect, while scheduling ongoing treatments with a naturopath in Calgary. He returned to work late in the fall of 2017, ambitious, full of life and with great respect for all that surrounded him.

At the first National Sales Meeting after his return, the company asked Terri if he would share a speech with his company. They all had been rooting for him and were equally amazed with the success that Terri had had beating Stage IV Pancreatic Cancer as they had for his work ethic. They requested that he share some of his insight. Terri felt honored to give a speech, but when he approached the podium nerves set in. Looking into the audience at his colleagues, managers and directors, he felt so privileged to be working for Apotex, yet incredibly overwhelmed to verbalize his story in public.

"My wife is my healer," he began. "She trusted her instincts for the path we walked along, and here I am standing. We understand the severity of the death sentence I was given, but we chose to look past it: to believe. It was not always easy, but here I am on my path to health and wholeness." He continued by walking through the story of his treatment and thanked them for their immense support.

When Terri retold the story he had experienced, giant bubble tears welled up in the corner of my eyes. Without doubt it was the most incredible compliment he had ever given me. Of course, I was relentless in my search for the path I thought would save him, but he did the work. Terri persevered and never gave up. I welcome you to do the same. When the going gets tough, the tough get going.

I was so proud of Terri to speak to his company, and I knew then that Terri was not only going to heal, but also become an inspiration to many around the world. We are so happy to share our story not only to heal our hearts, but to speak the truth of the power within us. Sometimes overwhelming to acknowledge, it is all worth it.

We are eternally grateful for Apotex, not only for their support but for reminding Terri of his inspirational power and potential.

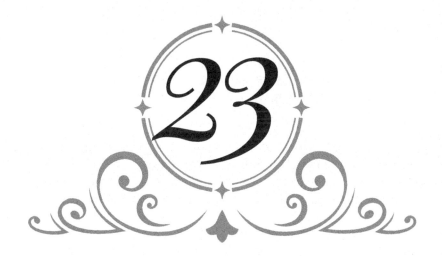

Chapter

BEACHFRONT BLISS

November was rainy and cool, and the snow had come and gone. Another blizzard was impending, and we were looking forward to our celebratory family trip to enjoy some beautiful weather. Sun, beach, and sand were on our bucket list for our family, and we only had to clear one important moment before we left.

November 25th was the first CT Terri would have that would measure his response to the treatment with Dr. Kleef. As we parked the truck to walk in to see Dr. Wirasinghe and receive the results, I placed my hand on Terri's arm before he could get out of the vehicle.

"I believe that you are really okay, my love. I honestly, honestly do." I spoke the words and a single tear rolled down my cheek. Terri gently wiped it away with his free hand and said, "I know, baby. I believe it too."

We took a deep breath and held hands as we walked into the clinic. We took our seats in the waiting area and did our best to distract ourselves with food or travel magazines. It was not long before the nurse called for us and guided us to a waiting room.

Dr. Wirasinghe entered the room and asked us how we were doing. She was inquisitive to know how our treatment went in Austria, and she was very happy to see Terri looking so radiant and healthy. She printed out the CT, handed us a copy, and we followed along as she read the results.

It read as follows:

Nov 25 CT

Compared to CT of abdomen and pelvis May 10, 2017

Findings:

The previously seen innumerable hypoattenuating lesions seen throughout the liver have decreased in size compared to previous, most of which are difficult to discretely measure on today's examination. The previously noted largest hepatic metastasis seen within segment 2 medially measures approximately 1.5cm, decreased in size compared to previous, where it measured approximately 2.0 cm. The 2nd largest lesion previously seen in segment 4A now measures approximately 1.0cm, previously 1.9cm.

The previously demonstrated ill-defined hypoattenuating mass within the body of the pancreas is not discretely measurable on today's examination. The degree of upstream dilation of the pancreatic duct has decreased compared to previous, now measuring up to 4mm, previously up to 8mm. No new pancreatic masses are identified.
The previously noted mildly enlarged peripancreatic lymph nodes are no longer discretely measurable.

Previously noted nodularity within the peritoneum, particularly on the right has resolved.

The region of the one of the previously suspected peritoneal nodules, a diverticulum arising from the cecal basis noted. The hollow abdominal viscera are otherwise unremarkable.

Impression: Positive treatment response, with decrease in size of the patient's primary pancreatic adenocarcinoma, numerous hepatic metastases and peritoneal metastases.

A smile swept across Dr. Wirasinghe's face, and I hugged Terri. The tumor in his pancreas and lymph nodes were still gone, and his liver had responded incredibly well. Most of the twenty plus lesions were now *difficult to discretely measure,* and the two discernable lesions remaining had shrunk in size substantially.

We spoke with Dr. Wirasinghe for a few more minutes and then went for lunch to celebrate. We had hoped, prayed, visualized and pulled out every stop to hear this truth. Servers in the restaurant must have thought we were newlyweds as we held hands and stared into each other's eyes full of love and hope. Terri was oh-so-close to Cancer Free, and we were only six months into the journey. He was healthy and full of life and it felt like the most incredible gift.

Sun on our Faces

Arriving in Mexico, it was the evening and the air was warm and full of love and anticipation. Palm trees waved in the wind, and the sunset lit up the sky with luminescent colours. On the way to our hotel room, the kids decided they would take a plunge into the pool, even though they were still in their clothes. After all, it was gorgeously hot outside and the pool seemed to be the perfect place to be.

I shrugged my shoulders and thought, "Why not join them?" I laughed and screeched, "Coming in!"

The kids backed up as I made an epic splash, while Terri just shook his head in a fun and loving kind of way.

We swam around the whole pool before deciding to climb out. The weight of our clothes was feeling heavy, and luckily, we had a few layers on from being on the plane. We wrung out our sweaters and skipped the entire way to our room sharing giggles about our *Big Splash!*

Each Moment is so Precious

The week flew by, and we swam and ate and ate and swam. We swam and ate some more and ate and swam even more. To some our beach vacation may seem simplistic, but to us it was paradise. The moments of sharing nachos by the pool, playing 500 for hours with a football, and having underwater handstand competitions never seemed to get old. We found a sense of wholeness in the magical moments of simplicity.

On our second last evening, we booked dinner at a beachside restaurant in the middle of our resort. Surrounded by palm trees and pools, we had an opulent view of the ocean, warm breeze wafting through our hair as we ate dinner. It was an exceptional evening, and we were not only celebrating Terri's health that night, it was also an occasion to celebrate our tenth anniversary which was upcoming the following month. Of course, I had pleaded with Terri to renew our vows in a ceremony with a fancy dress and flowers, and he gracefully declined. Nonetheless, we took a moment to hold hands and renew our vows in a beautiful moment shared with our children.

"You are my angel," Terri began, "And I am thankful every day for you. We have welcomed two beautiful children into this world and overcome heartache and challenges together. There may be ups and downs, but you are my destiny. We are meant to be together. I loved you then, I love you now, and I will love you forever."

The kids looked at us expectantly, enjoying the moment and hanging on every word that was spoken. You could see them feel our hearts beaming; they felt the sincerity of the moment and the true value of our family.

I took a deep breath, composing what could possibly be as powerful as the words Terri had just spoken.

"From the moment I met you, I knew you would challenge me. As we grew in our path together, I knew we were meant for each other. You are the strongest, and most graceful man I know. You radiate with a sense of purpose I have never seen, and I will forever call you my own. You may call me your healer, but I call you my rock. You are my home, and I never want to be anywhere else. Thank you for my children, thank you for our family, and cheers to many, many more years. I love you to the moon and back."

The kids began to giggle once I spoke the moon comment and we all laughed. Terri kissed me, just long and passionate enough that the kids said, "Ewwwwwww," and began to roll their eyes. As we finished clinking our glasses together—like a perfectly timed moment in a movie, the waiter came over with a beautiful plate of dessert.

"Congratulations," he began, "It is our privilege to have you here to celebrate your anniversary."

We thanked him and took a picture of the artistically designed plate. *Happy Anniversary* was written in delicate chocolate, surrounded by delicious strawberries adorning the cheesecake.

As we all enjoyed the dessert, Terri and I took the opportunity to tell the kids the story of our wedding. What a glorious night that had been! As I spoke, it felt as though the same magic danced in the air.

———————————◆———————————

A Day in Heaven

On December 29th, 2007, Terri and I became husband and wife. It was a beautiful winter wedding: reception room decorated with Christmas Trees, and hundreds of snowflakes hung from the ceiling. I wore fur boots under my dress for outdoor pictures in the snow, and our wedding party of sixteen carried us through the day with laughs and encouragement. It was the most magical day of my life, and I felt like a princess. I was so honoured to hold Terri's hand and proudly proclaim our vows that we were ready to be united. We had scripted our own words of love and were passionate about sharing them with each other. Terri adapted his a little at the last minute and started off like this:

"Well…. We all know that the cornerstone of a good marriage is punctuality!"

The entire congregation burst out laughing, and our wedding party could not help but bust a gut. You see, everything had gone smoothly at first, until my wedding dress broke. Yes, it broke. There are pictures of me lying on our bed as my bridesmaids sewed me into my dress! This was irony at its best as Terri's only request for me was to be punctual. A broken dress threw a wrench into that plan, and we arrived at the church almost an hour late.

Because he is such an incredible man, Terri did not spend time fuming or worrying. Rather, he entertained the audience and pretended to escape the church by running through the aisles and attempting to climb out of the windows. His groomsmen chased him to keep the excitement going, and before he knew it, I had arrived and the ceremony could begin.

The day was like a dream come true, and I will cherish it forever in my heart. We enjoyed family, friends, dancing and celebrating. Holding hands and knowing we had made the commitment to be together forever was more special than words can describe.

What is Normal?

Once we returned from Mexico, we settled back into a routine. Our kids were back at school, I was studying for my exams to become a Certified BodyTalk Practitioner, and Terri went back to work. It is interesting how focusing on the normality of life brought so much peace to our household. Terri's treatments had slowed, and we were in awe of how life had brought us to this point.

Imagine if we all altered our perception, just a little, to appreciate the day-to-day activities. If we could change our thinking from them being mundane to captivating. That we do not *have* to do something, but rather that we *have the opportunity* to accomplish something. Our routine was now filled with a different level of enthusiasm, and I knew that Terri and I were on a healing path. Not only was he going to be healed physically, but we were going to alter our destiny in its entirety.

If we allow ourselves to look for it, there is beauty in every moment. The more we begin to see it in the small things—a perfect four leaf clover, your child's dirty face from enjoying your home- cooked meal, your body's ability to exercise, or securing a new client at work, the more that our gratitude for the small things begins to envelop our hearts. Before we know it, all our small moments of gratitude encompass our entire day, and we can realize that we are not only changing our lives but living the truth of gratitude and the magic that lies within that experience.

Chapter

OH HOW TIME FLIES

Summarizing our past two years in one word is simple—beauty. The beauty that resonates in every day, the healing Terri has accomplished, and how incredibly the dynamic within our family unit has changed. We began to communicate with The Pancreatic Cancer Awareness Society of Canada to introduce them to the healing success that Terri has accomplished.

Recalling the beginning of our journey, the only option that was available in Canada for Terri was chemotherapy. We did not choose full-dose chemotherapy as an option, but we still maintained a connection with Dr. Scot Dowden, our oncologist in Canada. We saw him after every CT Scan, and after we reviewed the May 2018 CT, we had a very interesting and powerful conversation.

We were anticipatory of what the CT results would be, as Terri had travelled back to Austria again for one month of treatment in February 2018. He intended to go for only one week to receive the dose of immunotherapy he was unable to have in the fall of 2017 due to high liver enzymes, however once he arrived, we made the decision, in accordance with Dr. Kleef's recommendation, that it would be beneficial for Terri to undergo another round of treatment. He stayed for one month and doubled up on treatments. In that time, he had two doses of immunotherapy and went through fever week a second time. Mary travelled with him to keep him company. They were unable to adjust to the time change on this trip and were so appreciative that the Olympics were on. They kept the pair of them entertained for hours in the middle of the night!

The CT results from May 7, 2018 outlined the following:

CT Scan May 7/2018

Findings in Abdomen and Pelvis:

Liver; The previously seen hepatic metastases have further regressed in size and only faintly visible on today's study. Specifically, the lesion in segment 2 laterally near the dome is not well appreciated though this could be based on cardia motion artifact. A hypodense nodule with overlying capsular retraction measuring 5mm is stable. No new hepatic lesions are confidently detected. Hepatic and portal venous vasculature remains patent.

Pancreas: Again, seen is atrophy of the mid pancreatic body extending into the tail, similar to the prior study. The main pancreatic duct in this region remains mildly dilated at 4mm, stable. No peripancreatic fluid collections of stranding seen. No peripancreatic lymphadenopathy.

My visceral instincts told me at this moment that Terri was clear. I had always known that we would never be given a true *all-clear* diagnosis but had always trusted that Terri would be healed. I also believed that his healing would have a profound impact on our lives, and on the lives of so many around the world. The next words that Dr. Dowden spoke reiterated that feeling perfectly, "I have seen the incredible success you have had with immunotherapy in Austria," he began, "And I would like to see if we can get the process started here." Dr. Dowden was revered in Western Canada for pushing the boundaries of treatment, always wanting to offer innovative treatments to his patients.

The conversation continued and Dr. Dowden explained that Terri would have to go through a few tests, and if he met certain parameters, then Dr. Dowden could gain approval to have immunotherapy prescribed for him here in Canada.

We left the appointment, and I looked at Terri, a massive grin sweeping across my face.

"What's that all about?" he asked.

"I knew it," I said. "I knew it from day one. I trusted that not only were you going to be okay, but that you would have a huge impact on Pancreatic Cancer. Having immunotherapy prescribed for you here, in Canada, is changing the face of treatment options. Count on you to want to be the poster boy for Pancreatic Cancer!" I poked him in the side as a soft tickle, and he whacked my hand away with a *Stop it!*

It was so true. Here he was changing the face of history. Dr. Dowden received approval for Terri to receive immunotherapy, and we applied for coverage.

A New Perspective

To avoid repetition, we have not included every CT. However, there is one other that needs to be discussed. Once again, in August 2018, Terri and I were holding hands preparing to walk into Dr. Wirasinghe's office and receive our results. We were not seeing her on this day, but another doctor in the office, and although we enjoyed seeing Dr. Wirasinghe, every physician and staff member in the clinic always provided exceptional service and care to us.

It was a morning appointment, and we picked up a coffee and green tea before we headed in to the office. Strolling back to the clinic, I grabbed Terri's arm and stopped him in his tracks. Almost causing his tea to spill, he gave me a half-glare, half- perplexed look.

"I need to tell you something," I calmly asserted. It was a feeling in my heart, a feeling oh-so-bold that I was not sure I was brave enough to share.

"What is it? We are going to be late and need to get into the clinic." Terri spoke quickly, as being late was his nemesis.

"Well," I stumbled trying to get the words out quickly. "I have always known that you will never be given the all-clear. That it will be in our hearts to trust. I believe the moment is here. I know it. I know you are clear. I believe the cancer is gone. I feel it in my bones; my instincts are compelling me to tell you this…. and…." I hesitated for a moment and bowed my head, not sure Terri would believe me, "Since day one my primary Vision Board in MindScape has been a picture of our family celebrating you being cancer free. That Vision Board collapsed—it is gone. It is only gone because I believe and truly know, that you are cancer-free."

Terri grinned, half-processing but not really listening as he was focused on being on time for the appointment.
The CT results read as follows (in summary):

There are no definite enlarged lymph nodes identified within the mediastinum, hila or bilateral axillary regions. A Port-A-Cath is in satisfactory position.

Tiny hypodensities are present within the liver. Subcapsular lesion segment VII/VIII is stable, measuring up to 6mm. Segment II lesion is not well seen. Other small hypodensities appear stable. The spleen appears unremarkable. Again, within the pancreas is atrophy of the mid pancreatic body with mild dilation of the pancreatic duct, measuring up to 4mm. Bilateral adrenal glands appear unremarkable. Both kidneys demonstrate no worrisome abnormalities.

There it was—our truth. Who knows if the hypodensities in the liver were cancerous? We had to trust. I did. The work was there, and the proof was there. Terri Mah was on a journey to impeccable health, and quite likely had just arrived.

On the global scale of reviewing our lifetime, Terri and I have always felt the desire and drive to help others. Now we were gaining so much deep insight into our lives through his healing; I often wondered whether this was all part of the plan. It was sometimes difficult to be appreciative of watching Terri endure Stage IV Pancreatic Cancer, but as we grew more confident in our knowledge of BodyTalk and MindScape, we understood that this life is not about learning to accept reality but rather focusing on our incredible ability to create it.

We walked through the fire and changed our entire lives. In all honesty, it was no coincidence that we found Dr. Kleef, the perfectly suited oncologist for our needs. We all hold him in such high respect, and his innovative treatment plan is a crucial part of how our perceptions of what cancer treatment *should* look like shifted. Our priorities, perceptions, and moments of truth were altered. Our love for the mundane became inherent, and our appreciation for life so abundant. We were receiving calls— sometimes daily, sometimes weekly, and through Terri's story we were helping to offer hope. As Alanis Morrissette said it best, "Isn't that ironic?"

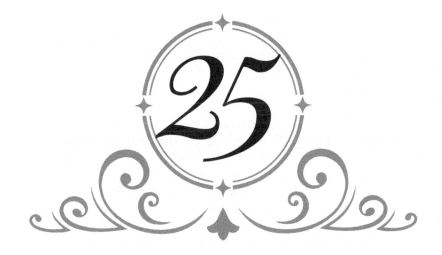

Chapter

PEEK-A-BOO I'M BACK

Life has a way of keeping you on your toes. Before you can praise overcoming one obstacle, another may rear its head. If you commit to evolving, time and again obstacles can be viewed as new doors for opportunity and growth. Just recently, we were faced with having to revisit our intentions once again.

Terri started to have back pain, and we blamed it on our mattress. After a number of nights, he would rotate to one of the kid's beds and still not sleep soundly, his back pain not diminishing. It was not the mattress causing the discomfort. I regularly was in touch with Dr. Dowden to see where we were with regards to the status of having immunotherapy covered, and now took the opportunity to request a CT scan for Terri as well. He pleasantly obliged, and Terri headed into the clinic.

The CT was scheduled for the end of September 2019, and we met with Dr. Wirasinghe to receive the results. Terri had had a CT earlier in the year, in March, when he was not feeling well after a trip to Mexico, and the results were still great. I had no anticipation of this being any different, and I certainly did not walk into the clinic emotionally prepared for the news we were about to receive.

Like a routine that we were oh-too-familiar with, Dr. Wirasinghe printed off the CT results and handed them to us for review. We were appreciative of how wonderful she was with us, and we know in our hearts we found the best GP in Calgary for our family. She has always been responsive, dedicated, and willing to accommodate us and our needs. There were multiple letters and forms we had requested for her to complete over the past two years, and she always completed them without hesitation. I wish she could take on a million patients because I would refer to her the entire city of Calgary.

As she handed us the document, I did not see the tenacious smile on her face this time. Instead it was replaced with perplexity, bundled with concern and curiosity.
The CT results illustrated the following:

CT Scan Sept 27/2019

Findings in Abdomen and Pelvis:

Liver: At the time of original diagnosis in 2017, there were greater than 20 hypoattenuating hepatic lesions. On today's evaluation, there are slightly larger and more conspicuous hypoattenuating hepatic lesions present when compared to April 2, 2019.

For example, there is a 1.2 cm in the right hepatic lobe near the dome (axial image 12) which previously was only at most 0.4 cm and more ill-defined than currently.

There is a 0.9cm more conspicuous hepatic segment 2 lesion, as well as a 0.7 cm lesion straddling hepatic segments 4A/8.

There is a 0.9cm lesion in segment 4, inconspicuous previously. There is a 1.3cm subcapsular lesion in segment 6. As well as an adjacent 0.8cm lesion and 1.1cm lesion more inferiorly.

Other tiny hypoattenuating lesions superiorly in the right lobe are unchanged.

Pancreas: The primary pancreatic lesion previously noted in the body is not conspicuous by CT. The appearance of the pancreas is unchanged from recent studies, with atrophy and duct dilation in the distal body and tail. There is slightly more prominent but nonspecific fat stranding in the pancreatic adrenal retroperitoneal fascia on the left.

Lymph nodes: Small superior peripancreatic node measures 0.6cm compared with 0.4 cm previously. Slightly more conspicuous but small sub centimeter lymph nodes with some surrounding fat stranding at the base of the SMA mesentery, with largest node measuring 0.6cm. SMA and SMV remain patent. Splenic vein remains patent. There is also a new prominent gastrohepatic region node measuring 1.0cm. There is also a worrisome increasing 0.8cm peripancreatic node.

Impression: Increase in size and number of hypoattenuating hepatic lesions since April 2019 is very worrisome for recurrent/ progressive hepatic metastatic disease.

Increase in size of multiple small lymph nodes in the peripancreatic region and base of the SMA mesentery. These are concerning for possible metastases as well.

The primary pancreatic lesion is not visible by CT, unchanged from recent prior, with stable atrophy and duct dilation of the distal body and tail of the pancreas.

Sadly, we were familiar enough with these terms and reviewing CT scans that Dr. Wirasinghe did not have to sugar coat what she was reading. She was calm and patient, and her message was clear— we needed to get in to see Dr. Dowden to review where we were at with immunotherapy and potentially other treatment options.

I lost my breath, and my head felt fuzzy. "Could this truly be happening?" I thought. We have come so far, and here we are again. One step forward, twenty steps back? My mind raced in a circle, and I barely noticed Dr. Wirasinghe kindly dismiss herself from the room. I lost track of time, my vision came back into focus to see Terri's hand ready to pull me off the chair and get us out of the clinic.

Over the following days, we walked in a daze and talked in a haze. We felt that overwhelming pressure of here we go again—not wanting to share the news and go through the motions. Not wanting to re-evaluate treatment options, and surely not wanting to believe that we had been wrong about Terri beating this obstacle. There was absolutely no way that that was true. There was just more work for us to do.

Apotex was incredibly supportive again; without hesitation, Terri's manager, Bill Krzysik, went above and beyond to make sure Terri was able to take time off work, and that his territory would be covered proficiently. Terri and Bill started work together at Apotex and had become close friends over the years. His swiftness and level of respect for Terri was above and beyond, and Terri was entirely appreciative. Again, we were at a loss of words Terri working for such an incredible organization.

We assessed whether Terri would travel back to Austria, and how we would break the news to our children. In the end, we simply told them, "You know the cancer in daddy's liver is not quite gone, so he is taking a little bit of time to work on it." That explanation seemed to suffice, and the optimism remained in their eyes. We hoped that we were hiding the fear in ours.

Other than fever week, Terri determined we could do immuno-therapy here in Canada now that it was approved by Dr. Dowden, and the other essential treatments with his naturopath, Dr. Matt Pyatt. Dr. Pyatt specializes in cancer treatments and works diligently to bring in innovative options. Terri had been seeing him off and on outside of his time in Austria, and Dr. Pyatt, by no coincidence, even knew Dr. Kleef and worked by the same principles he did. Terri immediately began seeing Dr. Pyatt for IV Vitamin-C and alpha-lipoic treatments while we determined the next steps in our action plan.

Over the past two and a half years, our understanding of the power of the mind has deepened immensely. We have also added meditation to our repertoire of our BodyTalk and MindScape strategies. I will never forget the first time I tried meditating; it shook me to the core. As I had experienced with numerous BodyTalk and MindScape experiences, I felt knocked off my feet in such a positive way. I calmed my ego and welcomed another opportunity to grow and develop. My strength and drive to share this with Terri was perpetuated with baby steps. At first, I had to introduce it to him with mild conversations, texts of screenshots captivating motivational quotes, and playing a meditation while in his presence. I was instantly drawn to the teachings of Dr. Joe Dispenza and knew how much of an impact they were going to have on my life.

As we faced this obstacle again, I wondered what was needing to be accomplished. Once the fear passed for both of us, our optimism resurfaced, and we were back in focus with a plan. He considers me his healer, I thought to myself. I trusted my instincts then, and I was going to trust them again now.

Terri knew he needed to dig deeper. As soon as he received the news of the CT scan, he prepared himself to go further into the shadows. After all, in Eastern Medicine the consciousness of the liver is anger and resentment, and that was a powerful realization for Terri. Now so aware of how the bodymind complex functions as one, he recognized that there was unhinged emotion stored in his liver, and likely elsewhere, that needed to be released. How was he going to do this?
He continued with Eastern Medicine treatments at the naturopath, maintaining his use of Celebrex and Co-Enzyme Q10, and kept his

routine of accessing his MindScape every evening when he put one of the kids to bed (we happily alternated evenings with each kiddo). We were still awaiting the approval of immunotherapy to be covered for us here in Canada, and in addition, he continued frequent BodyTalk sessions. However, God and the Universe was prompting us to do more: to dig deeper, come out brighter. It was no coincidence that I had started down the path of meditation. He had begun to try the occasional meditation, but often used it more as an excuse to nap than to transform.

My instincts were guiding me down the path, loudly and clearly. As his healer, what could I possibly provide Terri that would take his growth to the next level? Why, a Dr. Joe Dispenza Advanced Meditation Workshop of course! The walls went up and Terri bucked and bashed, stating that it was my dream to attend the workshop, and he did not need to go. I knew it was meant to be when the workshop was sold out, and a kind and desperate email to Joe Dispenza's staff was promptly returned with a spot reserved for Terri in the Cancun workshop December 2019. Oh, how things align! There are no coincidences. Trust those instincts!

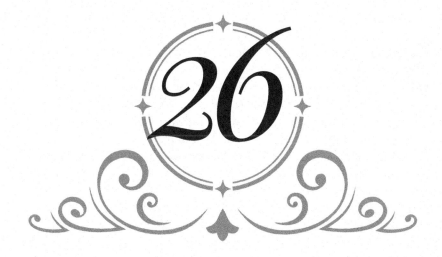

Chapter

MEDITATION MOTIVATION

The sun rises and sets every day, and like clockwork it begins the opportunity for a fresh start. The colours of the event paint the sky brilliantly and leave visions of our future dancing in the distance. We watched the sunset time and again as we passed our week in Mexico. December was humid and warm, just nice enough to take the chill off the water, and not too hot that frequent shade cover was required. The kids and I were accompanied by great friends from Saskatoon, and we passed the days frolicking in the sand, snorkeling for sea creatures, and playing endless games of football.

We always cherished family vacations, but the agenda of Mexico, December 2019 was slightly different for us. We had a three-bedroom condo at our favourite resort near Playa De Carmen, and we shared it with Kristi and Andrew. Their boys, Lucas and Logan, were close to the ages of our kids and were always able to entertain one another. That made it a little easier as my pool entertaining skills began to run dry long before the enthusiasm of the children.

It was an enjoyable trip, days turning into nights, and nights back into sunlit mornings. We would swim, eat, play and await news as Terri would roll in at bedtime from many hours away at the Dr. Joe Dispenza retreat at a neighbouring resort. We would hang on his words, as he would share the details of the interesting people he would meet from around the world, the power of your breath, and the enlightening experiences he would have from four- or five-hour meditations. He marveled at how Dr. Joe was able to keep a group of well over a thousand people entertained with dialogue, experiences and meditations. I marveled at the incredible effort my husband was putting into the workshop. Only days earlier, while still in Canada, he was adamant that I should take his place and that it was my dream to attend. It certainly was that, and I will be on a plane in 2020 to experience a workshop for myself.

The question is this—Is a desire for change something you really, truly want? Your dreams cannot be dictated by others in your life; they need to come from a place of your truth to manifest your destiny. I knew Terri would come on board to attend the workshop. I could not physically go in his presence, and this experience was not for me. I knew it in my heart, and I trusted my instincts were spot on. I also knew that his ego was trying to protect him, his body exerting physical symptoms, and his shifting occurring from the moment he committed to attending.

It was a big leap for Terri to attend. God guided us to this point with the CT showing a negative turn and forcing Terri to dig deeper if he truly wanted to be cancer free. As a bystander, the most profound experience of all is to watch what heals alongside the physical cancer dissipating: the improvements in our marriage, new perspectives on what is the meaning of life, how to parent our children, and how to disengage from that which is unimportant—it has been fascinating. In a simple dialogue, Terri explained to me the realization he had during a meditation. When asked to confront something that was problematic in his life, a conversation appeared to him like a vision. It was one where we were arguing, and my disagreement stirred up a level of annoyance within Terri. This is completely normal within a marriage, but something we have been working on for a long time. It has been improving, and while I work on letting go of control, Terri has been focusing on how easily he gets frustrated and annoyed with me. He was telling me this story, and I waited with bated breath and curiosity to hear what the solution was for him. I was assuming that it would be an adept and positive strategy, as he was deep in a meditative state, well within his subconscious mind. I would be lying if I did not admit that some fear crept into my heart. Would he say that I needed to change? Of course, we all need to grow and develop, but my ego prepared me for an attack. It was a small moment in time, at the cafeteria of an airport, but even reliving it now brings tears to my eyes. He continued with the story of how he should handle things if we are disagreeing, and he looked at me with more love in his eyes than I have ever seen.

"I will just take your hand," he said calmly, "And ask you why you are feeling that way or how you think we should handle the situation." Him touching my hand in that moment felt so different, so innocent and reminiscent of a first date, that I did not need any more words about how the week had transformed him from the inside out. The way he looked at me was so full of love and gratitude, it was overwhelming. My heart sang for our future in that moment, not just a cancer free future, but one of a deepened relationship. One that can stand the test of time when kids leave the house, and we are empty nesters with a deck of cards. In our twelve years of marriage thus far, we have faced our tribulations, and instead of pulling us apart every challenge has brought us closer together. We may not always like each other, and understand that is completely normal as well, but we certainly love and respect each other. Now, through all the work we have done in the past two and a half years healing Terri's cancer, we also healed our marriage. In my meditations, I am working to let go of so many old hurts and traumas, and Terri is doing the same. What is left is a new sense of appreciation—not only for us as individuals, but for our marriage and for our children.

That moment at the airport was another pivotal moment for our story, one I will cherish in my heart forever. The warmth of his hand sent tingles up my arm, and my heart felt as though it was going to explode. The love in his eyes was so genuine, if there was nothing else—I could thank Dr. Joe for, it would be the next step of transformation in our marriage. I knew, however, that there was so much that Terri learned and experienced in the Advanced Retreat. Some of it I will hear about, as the stories trickle in over time, and some transformations may be forgotten as they were released into the quantum field while Terri was in a meditative state. I am not bothered either way, as meditation is now a way of life for us, a daily routine, and sometimes the transformations do not need words attached to them. They might just be evident with the touch of a hand.

Why Meditate?

Through the words in this book, through our stories of healing, Terri and I discovered first-hand how accessing the subconscious part of our mind is where we are capable of true change. Working through barriers, traumas, energies and fears do affect our personal health. It is all connected. Just as MindScape is a powerful tool to access your subconscious, and one both Terri and I use daily, meditation is another tool to have in your repertoire. Simply put—meditation is another method we can use to access the mind's operating system. It can be a resource anytime, anywhere, for anyone. You just need to be a willing participant.

From the beginning of my meditative journey, I was gravitationally drawn to the work of Dr. Joe Dispenza. He has an incredible world-wide following and has impacted the lives of millions in epic ways.

He summarizes his work and the impact of how meditation can change your life in the following passage, speaking on the Law of Attraction the Quantum Way in an interview with Lilou Mace:

In order to manifest your dreams, it requires a Clear Intention; an Intention is a Vision, a Possibility. The moment you say, what would it be like to Be Healthy, what would it be like to Be Wealthy, what would it be like to Have a New Home, what would it be like to Have a Great Job? And you get this Idea in Your Mind; that's Intention. Then you write down the details, okay I want to travel around the world, I want to have great benefits, I want to work with really cool people, I want to have a chance to be creative, and you list all of those individual elements to fortify your dream; the more clear on those details, the more your brain begins to work in new ways; any time you make your brain work differently, you're changing your mind. Now, the moment you get inspired and you begin to feel what it would be like to live in that future, your body is getting a Chemical Sampling and Emotional Sampling, it's getting a Taste of the Future. That should be the new addiction, but it doesn't mean you try, there's no wishing, there's no hoping; hope is a beggar. It has to then Open your Heart, you have to move into an Elevated State. This place, Heart Center, is the Center of Creation. So as an example, in our advanced workshops, we start every Meditation where people begin to become Heart-Centered, they place their attention in their Heart, they begin to breathe through that Center, they begin to radiate that energy of gratitude, of joy; and if they do it enough times, we've measured this; the Field around their body is enhanced, they're producing a Magnetic Field that's connecting them to something greater. When they have that Magnetic Field now, it is amplified because this is the Center that causes the Field around your body to move up to 9 meters wide. The antithesis of that is when you're angry or you're aggressive or you're hating or you're judging or you're fearful, you're drawing from this Field and you're turning it into Chemistry and the Field and your body shrinks and now you're More Matter and Less Energy, More Particle and Less Wave, you're Separate from Possibility, you're Separate from the Field. But when you begin to open that Heart, you're amplifying your Energy, you're amplifying that Magnetic Field; then that Energy is Carrying the Thought, Carrying the Intention. And when you combine that, you are Broadcasting a Signature into the Field, and whatever you Broadcast into the Field is your experiment with Destiny. So then, most people then walk around in their life angry and upset and frustrated and suffering and victimized; basically, they're Broadcasting that Signature into the Field, and they wonder why their prayers aren't answered because, in order to do this properly, you have to get up as if your prayers are already answered. So we don't do our Meditations in the work that we teach our students how to do this, pray to have their prayers answered; we teach them how to get up as if their prayers are already answered because now the Signal has made it into the body, Signals made it into the Field, Mind is changed, the Gene has been Signaled, and every single day, they're knocking on that Genetic door; Why? Because a Gene makes a Protein, and the body must physically be prepared for the event, otherwise it can't have it. So, once they understand it, then they say, okay I'm going to teach my body Emotionally what it's going to feel like before it occurs. Now, what is the Emotion you would feel if you had your dream come true? Pretty excited, joyful, inspired, incredible gratitude. What is gratitude? The Emotional Signature of Gratitude means, the Event has Already Occurred; and if you can hold on to that Emotional State of Gratitude, your body is living in that Future in the Present moment, and that's when we begin to see the Miracles Happen.

Terri's Miracle

Terri does not like the word miracle. To him it implies that the cancer leaving his body just happened, some random event as rare as it is occurring in the first place. Terri knows the work—the days, the hours, the thought processes, the change in lifestyle, the techniques and shadows he has thrown himself into. All of this work has been to come out the other side healthy, whole, and cancer-free. To us reading this, and to those who have witnessed it in person, it is a miracle. It's not a tiny miracle, but a miracle of epic proportions that leaves some scratching their heads and others wanting to learn every detail of how we accomplished it. The thing is this, and we have alluded to this time and again— Terri did it all. The all encompassed physical treatments and guidance from Dr. Kleef coupled together with the deep internal work Terri was committing to daily. It was not always pretty facing the shadows, and we will never be able to provide a ratio of what worked best, or which impacted him the quickest. All we can do is share the story. The lesson is this—as Dr. Joe says, the miracles happen when you accomplish all that deep work to truly experience the emotional signature of gratitude. It is difficult and wonderful work all at the same time. Our egos may try to block us, but if you are truly ready for change and healing do your research. Find the options that exist in the world for you.

If you have cancer or chronic illness, reach out, go to Dr. Kleef's clinic. Explore BodyTalk, try MindScape, and just as important, start meditating. Attend a Dr. Joe Dispenza Advanced Retreat. It will all change your life, in more ways than you could ever dream of imagining. You must get out of your own way. If you start feeling like you do not have the time to meditate, or find time for that treatment, take a deep breath. If you wonder why that future may be for someone else but not for you, or believe I am not strong enough, take a deep breath. Whatever the thoughts may be, thank your ego (I still love to use *Nice Kitty* to calm it down) for trying to protect you and then get to work.

No coincidences exist, and we must trust our instincts as our internal compass. Terri experienced many of these moments during his week at the Dr. Joe workshop. Once we start opening our eyes, truly listening to what others are saying, observing our own internal realities, and widening our focus, more moments will come: moments of change, moments of growth and moments of miracles. Terri's miracle is that his destiny is to be cancer free, to change how others view Stage IV Pancreatic Cancer, and for us to be able to use this book to provide inspiration.

———————————◆———————————

All in a Moment

There were many meditations at the weeklong Advanced Retreat. Terri would leave some mornings before 6am, and others as early as 4am. For a man who had meditated less than fifty times before the workshop, once he was in, he was in. Dr. Joe made the experience so captivating, and the meditations so enthralling. Terri, who two months previous was not able to last more than twenty minutes was now successfully meditating for upwards of five hours. He felt incredible transformations, many of which will unravel over the years to come.

There was only one meditation where Terri had to excuse himself to use the washroom. He just found it physically impossible to last the duration, so he exited the theater. The only unfortunate part was that once one left the meditation, understandably the doors were locked, and re-entry was not permitted. Passing the time in the hallway, Terri began talking with a lady who needed to excuse herself as well. Considering herself clairvoyant, they shared each other's stories, and she then offered Terri a piece of her wisdom. She explained that he was on the healing path, and that he would be cancer free, and he just had to plug in the right information. When he questioned her on what exactly that meant, she could provide no further details, but just told Terri he would know. At the meditation the next morning, there was a moment when Terri had a surge of energy, and he knew it was time for the positivity and healing energy to be plugged in. He envisioned a computer stick with all the healing information he needed plugging into his frontal cortex. Just as he did this, Dr. Joe explained in the meditation that they were to envision turning the radio on and tuning into the right frequency. Terri said this was a monumental moment for him—as he felt as though he picked up on Dr. Joe's information, and that there was no coincidence between the lady in the hallway, installing the plug-in, and Dr. Joe providing instruction that, to Terri, had aligned perfectly with the healing action he had just taken.

Throughout the duration of the week, there were a variety of meditations and strategies offered. The intention of this chapter is not to outline them all, but rather to give another reminder of the healing and abundance that can occur if you are willing to do the work. Noteworthy, however, is that pre-workshop you can apply for a group healing. Not everyone is chosen, but if you are, it is an epic moment. The positive and transformative energy of the masses of people intending on improving themselves is already dramatic, but in a group healing the energy is focused entirely on you.

When I completed the application for Terri—and registered him for the workshop, my instincts said he was going to be chosen. That is why we were drawn to the workshop; that was the healing he needed as part of his destiny. A few days into the workshop, they let Terri know that he was, in fact, chosen for a group healing on the last day of the retreat. I wept tears of joy, poolside onlookers wondering what on my phone could possibly be so captivating.

The last day came. Terri had no idea who was going to be involved as he lay down and prepared himself to receive the healing. It came as no surprise that the clairvoyant lady he spoke with in the hallway, out of over one thousand attendees, was one of less than ten healers there. Terri experienced the intensity of the group healing, with all love and attention directed towards him; subsequently, he released powerful amounts of emotion. He felt lighter in some ways and some ways transformed so deeply it will never be seen on a physical level. His chance meeting with her was no coincidence, and whether we see her as an angel or just a wonderfully bright spot in the experience, her final words as they finished the healing were that Terri's cancer was gone.

——————————————◆———————————————

A New Outlook

If you asked us at the beginning of this journey if either of us had meditated, we both would have sheepishly giggled, shook our heads and thought it was a silly man's game. We understood that it could calm your mind, but that there were certainly not enough hours in a day to find time to entertain the idea. At the workshop, Terri meditated more in one week than we had in our lifetimes. He is already wanting to attend another Dr. Joe Advanced Workshop, brings friends, and tells me it is a must on my list for 2020. Meditation with our kids will become part of our routine, and it will be amazing to watch new opportunities emerge, and barriers fall for them because really, at the end of the day, where do the barriers come from? We create them ourselves through our conditioning and our perceptions of ourselves and the world around us. The sky is not the limit, only our beliefs systems are. Dream big, heal big, let all these tools guide your way. Throw in a Dr. Joe workshop when you can—not only is it abundantly rewarding and eye opening, it is an experience that is literally almost impossible to categorize.

If we all as humanity collectively worked on changing our consciousness, all taking the time, opportunity and willingness to explore deeper—what a world this would be. Not only would we be able to transform ourselves, but our entire would be changed... How magical!

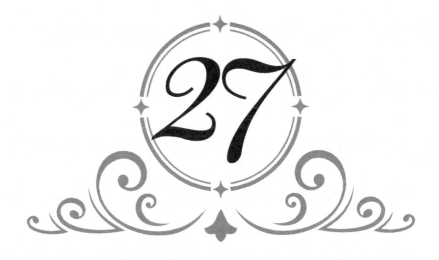

Chapter

ONE IN 10 BILLION

The awakening can happen at any time. It can take you by surprise, day or night, young or old. For some it may happen with a moment's effort, and for others it may be years of work. The transformations we have seen in our own family in a short couple of years leads me to believe in incredible possibilities. I am full of gratitude and anticipation to see what the future holds for us.

There was a moment during this journey that I wanted to put transformation to the test. It was not a feat as grandiose as conquering cancer, but it was an obvious change. I had a large mole on the right side of my cheek by my ear. It had changed shape during pregnancies and being slightly malformed it often worried me. I worked on it daily with BodyTalk, thanked it for being there and welcomed it to leave as it was no longer needed. Within a couple of months, it diminished greatly, and then one day flaked and fell off. It is completely gone!

It reminded me of a time when I was a child and had a wart on my pinkie finger. My mom never took me to the doctor, she just gave me similar instructions as I used for my mole. As a child, I never questioned my mom or thought that her instructions were strange by any means. My wart disappeared—and never returned. I thanked it every day for being there, and kindly excused it. I had forgotten that memory until we began this BodyTalk journey, and it reminds me how incredible God and the Universe really is. Over thirty some years ago, I was implementing techniques from the power of the mind.

I did not think at that moment that God was guiding my path towards some level of enlightenment or an understanding of how to trust the journey. All I knew was that my mom, who I adored and cherished for her wisdom, was providing simple advice on how to solve a problem. I use these strategies now with my children and hope that with all we have learned it will have as profound of an impact on their lives as it has ours. Without doubt, the transformation Terri and I have been through will greatly affect their destinies in a magnificent way.

We all have visions within our hearts. Sometimes they may be big, and others may be small. Often, we shy away from our visions, not understanding our true powers and capabilities to accomplish them. We keep our visions hidden deep within our soul, and although alive to us, they are often invisible to others. Take the opportunity to share them! Believe in them, shout from the rooftop that you are going to heal, achieve the goals you only dreamed of, and shine for the world.

Sometimes, we are lucky enough that events will happen to help us realize those visions and achieve those potentials. You may bump into someone on the street who turns out to be the love of your life. A driver may crash into your parked car, and when it's being assessed you find out there was a major fault, so what initially seemed like bad luck could have actually saved your life. You might be diagnosed with terminal cancer, as Terri was. In the prime heat of the moment, it is so difficult to see why things are happening, especially when they cause pain and destruction. It took time for me to understand why my dad passed away, and it took a lot of hard work to see why Terri needed to go through Stage IV Pancreatic Cancer with all odds stacked against him.

Today we see that it had to happen to encourage us to reach our potential and bring our vision of helping others to fruition. We stand ready to share this book on the brink of a new decade, to show that we all have unlimited capabilities within us. As they say in Star Wars (this one is for Terri), "The power is within us."

We need to be brave enough to go through the events and obstacles, and doing the work to understand them. As Yung Pueblo says:

Healing—it is a process that requires repetition so that we can remove more and more of the heavy conditioning. The mind is like an ocean and normally we swim on the surface, but if we truly want to be free, we need to be brave enough to swim within the deep.

At this exact moment in time, we cannot yet proclaim that Terri is 100% cancer free as proven by a CT scan. In fact, and in all honesty, he faced a turn for the worse. Is it any coincidence that on the verge of this book being launched, he may be met with some resistance? His physical body may be experiencing pain right now, the first true time he has felt the angst of deep pain and nausea in his cancer journey. He is determined as ever to work through the layers of fear and anger that lie below and will heal again. Refreshing update, since time of writing, is that he has come through the worst of it and is continuing his healing journey with each passing day.

Terri Mah is a survivor and continues to show he will beat the odds, and we still believe this happened for a reason. We trust that God and the Universe has given us all we need—within us. Remember, have the strength to walk through the obstacles and witness powerful reform. Remember, the bodymind connection provides us tools and awareness into infinite possibilities of healing and growth. And remember, gratitude and love can transform all.

Trust that the power is within us! Trust your instincts, thank your ego for protecting you, and then take your opportunity. We can all learn from Terri's story. We can all be shining lights in the dark. We can all be diamonds in the rough. Without doubt, we can all be one in 10 billion. We wish you the best on your journey.

Made in USA - Kendallville, IN
1237081_9781777152727
02.22.2021 0837